SURGICAL PEARLS

D1367945

SURGICAL PEARLS

ROBERT A. KOZOL, MD

Associate Professor of Surgery
Wayne State University
Chief of Surgery
Veterans Administration Medical Center
Detroit, Michigan

DIANA L. FARMER, MD

Associate Professor
Division of Pediatric Surgery
University of California, San Francisco
San Francisco, California

STEVEN D. TENNENBERG, MD

Assistant Professor
Wayne State University School of Medicine
Director of Surgical Intensive Care Unit
Veterans Administration Medical Center
Detroit, Michigan

MICHAEL MULLIGAN, MD

Lecturer, Thoracic Surgery
Section of Thoracic Surgery
University of Michigan
Ann Arbor, Michigan

 F. A. DAVIS COMPANY • Philadelphia

F. A. Davis Company
1915 Arch Street
Philadelphia, PA 19103

Printed in Canada

Last digit indicates print number: 10 9 8 7 6 5 4 3 2 1

Acquisitions Editor: Robert W. Reinhardt
Developmental Editor: Bernice M. Wissler
Cover Designer: Louis J. Forgione

As new scientific information becomes available through basic and clinical research, recommended treatments and drug therapies undergo changes. The author(s) and publisher have done everything possible to make this book accurate, up to date, and in accord with accepted standards at the time of publication. The authors, editors, and publisher are not responsible for errors or omissions or for consequences from application of the book, and make no warranty, expressed or implied, in regard to the contents of the book. Any practice described in this book should be applied by the reader in accordance with professional standards of care used in regard to the unique circumstances that may apply in each situation. The reader is advised always to check product information (package inserts) for changes and new information regarding dose and contraindications before administering any drug. Caution is especially urged when using new or infrequently ordered drugs.

Library of Congress
Cataloging-in-Publication Data

Surgical pearls / Robert A. Kozol . . . [et al.].
   p.   cm.
  Includes index.
  ISBN 0-8036-0388-6 (alk. paper)
  1. Surgery Handbooks, manuals, etc.   I. Kozol, Robert A.
  [DNLM: 1. Surgery Handbooks.   WO 39 S9598 1999]
RD37.S88   1999
617—dc21
DNLM/DLC
for Library of Congress   99-22366
                                       CIP

Preface

Day one as a student or first-year resident on a surgical service may be intimidating. We wrote the introductory chapters of *Surgical Pearls* to ease this anxiety. They describe the members and functions of the surgical team, introduce operating room jargon and etiquette, and name and describe basic instruments and sutures. We also present mnemonics and boilerplates to help the novice to write admitting and post-operative orders.

The remainder (and most) of the book, however, covers the "meat and potatoes" of surgical diseases, discussing all major organ systems plus burns, transplants, and pediatric surgery. Our goal was to alert the novice to the most common or critical diseases affecting each system, with diagnostic tips and advice on the way each disease is usually treated. Along the way, "Pearls" of "must-know" information are highlighted, as are "Controversies" that may come up in the course of surgical rounds.

Surgical Pearls will not replace a textbook, but we hope that reading it at the start of the surgical rotation will contribute to the breadth of knowledge expected of both senior students and junior residents. They can fill in the details from larger books while continuing to carry this book for quick reference (it really does fit into a lab coat pocket!). We also hope that readers will find its prose more enjoyable to read than the lists, algorithms, and outlines of most other surgical paperbacks. An unread book teaches nothing.

ROBERT A. KOZOL
DIANA L. FARMER
STEVEN D. TENNENBERG
MICHAEL MULLIGAN

Contents

vii

1
PART

Getting Started

1
CHAPTER

Introduction To The Surgical Service

Most surgical training programs use a team approach to patient care. A typical team includes a Chief Resident (usually a fifth-year postgraduate) and any number of midlevel and junior residents. Most teams also include medical students. The team is commonly responsible for the care of patients belonging to 3 to 10 attending surgeons. Thus, the resident must learn the habits, likes, and dislikes of different surgeons.

THE SURGICAL DAY

A typical day on the surgical service begins early. Because most operating suites begin elective cases at 7:30 or 8:00 AM, surgeons must complete morning rounds before that time. On many surgical services, students are expected to have seen their patients before morning rounds with residents. A worklist, or "scut list," created by the resident team lists chores or tasks that must be completed during the day. The list may include dressings to be changed, IV lines to be placed, x-ray studies to be arranged, and other tasks.

When the Operating Room (OR) begins morning cases, most residents and students scrub on OR cases (patients

3

scheduled for operation). At least one resident and perhaps several students are designated as outpersons. The
outperson, or outman, is responsible for the work list. Different teams establish different customs to complete daily
progress notes in the chart and to do other daily tasks.

Rounds

Morning rounds and late afternoon or evening rounds
follow the day's OR work. These rounds are often teach-
ing rounds involving bedside visits to every patient on the
list. The success of such a surgical team is highly dependent on the organizational skills of the Chief Resident.

On rounds with more senior team members, the medical student may be expected to **present** his or her patients. If the patient is new, the student should present
pertinent history (here details may be important), physical findings, and laboratory and x-ray results. The student may then be asked about the diagnosis or differential diagnosis.

For patients who are not new to the surgical service,
students may be asked to give an update or progress re-
port. Note that the average student can regurgitate vital
signs and daily lab results, but the *superior* student can
follow these with a conclusion, such as that the patient
is getting better, is getting worse, or is stable.

Conferences

At some conferences, students are innocent bystanders.
At others, they are expected to participate. Participation
may include case presentation. At times, students are
asked to interpret x-rays. If you are asked to interpret x-
rays, stay calm and read films systematically:

- Start by identifying the films: for example, "This is
  a PA (posteroanterior) and lateral chest film" or
  "This is a CT scan of the abdomen."
- Do not jump to an obvious finding such as a pneu-
  mothorax or tumor mass.
- Systematically look at bony structures, soft tissues,
  and so on.
- Point out abnormal findings.

THE OPERATING ROOM

Entering the OR for the first time is somewhat analogous to traveling in a foreign country because the OR has its own culture. This culture includes its own fashions, rituals, habits, and unique language or, more specifically, terminology.

Most hospitals provide a **scrub orientation** to teach medical students how to scrub and how to observe sterile technique. Scrubbing involves the use of disinfecting soaps such as iodoforms (Betadine) and chlorhexidine. Sterile brushes and nail cleaners are stocked in plastic wrap at the scrub sinks.

Scrub Technique

Follow this technique for preoperative scrubbing:

- Unwrap a brush and wet down both forearms and hands with water and the soap of choice.
- After establishing a preliminary lather, use the plastic nail cleaner packaged with the brush to clean beneath all fingernails.
- Use the brush, covered with soap, to scrub each finger. Treat each finger as if it had four sides and scrub each of the four sides one by one until all 10 fingers have been scrubbed.
- Next scrub the palms and backs of the hands.
- Finally scrub the wrists and forearms to the elbow.

Most surgeons scrub from 5 to 10 minutes, depending on the case. If you finish too quickly, simply repeat the process. The scrub is finished with a rinse. To rinse, allow the water to run from your hands toward your elbows (theoretically from the cleanest area toward the dirtiest area).

With the scrub completed, proceed into the OR, pushing the door open with your back. Hold your hands up and away from your body, thus maintaining **sterile technique.** In the room, the scrub nurse will hand you a sterile towel. Dry your arms from hands to elbows (as with the rinse sequence). The scrub nurse will then gown and glove you. **PEARL: Once gowned and gloved, to avoid contaminating yourself, never touch your mask or drop your hands below your waist.**

Touching your mask, dropping your hands below your waist, or touching other nonsterile items in the room will necessitate regowning and gloving. Remember that your arms, hands, and anterior gown are *sterile*. Your back, head, and neck are not.

OR TEAM MEMBERS

In addition to the surgeon, residents, and students, there are several other key members of the OR team.

Circulating Nurse

The circulating nurse, or **circulator,** who is usually a registered nurse (RN), helps prepare the room for the operation, brings the patient into the operating room (OR), and comforts the patient. He or she may place on the patient such devices as a grounding pad for electrocautery, or inflatable boots or stockings to minimize the risk of deep venous thrombosis. The circulating nurse is also responsible for obtaining any other items or instrumentation required during the operation. After surgery the circulator facilitates moving the patient to the recovery area.

Scrub Nurse

The **scrub nurse** can be a nurse or a technician. This person's role includes gowning and gloving the surgical team. Most importantly, the scrub nurse prepares the instruments beforehand and passes them to the surgeon as they are called for. A talented scrub nurse can anticipate what will be needed before it is requested, thus cutting minutes from operating times and improving team efficiency.

Anesthetists

An individual operative case may require anywhere from no anesthesia personnel (straight local anesthetic by the surgeon) to an anesthesia team of three or four persons for complex operations such as open-heart surgery. Such a team frequently includes certified registered nurse anesthetists and anesthesiologists. Anesthesia residents and students may also be included. Anesthetists not only administer anesthetic agents but also monitor the patient for physiologic changes during the operation.

CONDUCT OF THE OPERATION

A member of the surgical team "preps" the region of the body to be operated on. Prepping involves the following:

- A 5- to 10-minute washing of the operative area with disinfecting soap (may involve hair removal).
- The surgeons drape the patient with sterile drapes made of paper or cloth.

After the incision is made, **exposure** of the operative field becomes important. Exposure involves positioning retractors (see Chapter 2) and moving organs to allow the operating surgeon an adequate field of vision. Students play an important role in the operation because they are frequently asked to hold retractors. During the operation, exposure is as critical as the actual surgical technique. Additional technical roles for students may include cutting sutures, simple skin suturing, and skin stapling.

During the scrub—and certainly during the operation—the student may be asked questions concerning anatomy or pathophysiology relating to that patient's disease. You should therefore identify your assigned case or cases for the next day and read about them the night before.

2
CHAPTER

Instruments and Sutures

The most important tools of the surgeon are instruments and sutures. Although there are thousands of hand-held instruments, familiarity with common instruments (Table 2–1) will suffice for the novice.

COMMON SURGICAL INSTRUMENTS

Scalpel

The scalpel, or "knife," is used for cutting skin and fascia. It may also be used for sharp dissection. Scalpel handles come in several lengths. The blades are disposable. A #10 blade is used for most major surgery. A #15 blade is commonly used for finer work and in cosmetic surgery (Fig. 2–1).

Hemostat

A hemostat is also known as a clamp. Hemostats are most commonly used for division and ligation of small blood vessels. They come in a variety of sizes from small "mosquitoes" to large Kelly clamps (Fig. 2–2).

Table 2–1. COMMON SURGICAL INSTRUMENTS

Instrument Type	Function
Scalpel (knife)	Incisions and sharp dissection
Hemostat (clamp)	Grasping small blood vessels for hemostasis
Suture scissors	Cutting suture
Tissue scissors (many types)	Sharp dissection
Needle holder	Holding needle for suturing
Retractor	Moving body wall or organs to gain exposure

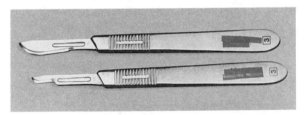

Figure 2–1. (*Top*) Scalpel with #10 blade, commonly used to open either chest or abdomen. (*Bottom*) Scalpel with #15 blade, used for finer work, such as excision of skin lesions.

Scissors

Scissors are used for dissection. There are many sizes and varieties of dissecting scissors. They are commonly named after surgeons, such as Metzenbaums and Mayos (Fig. 2–3).

Suture scissors are designed—you guessed it—to cut sutures.

Forceps

The two major types of forceps are the tweezers-type and the hemostat-shaped forceps (Fig. 2–4).

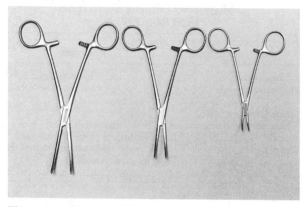

Figure 2–2. Hemostats (also known as clamps) come in three sizes. Shown left to right are the Kelly, Crile, and mosquito, also called a snap.

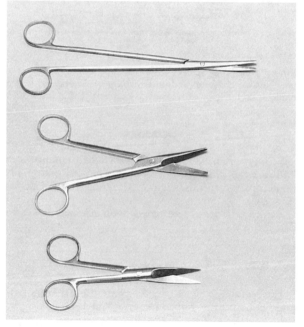

Figure 2–3. Dissecting scissors: Metzenbaum (*top*), Mayo (*center*), and straight suture (*bottom*).

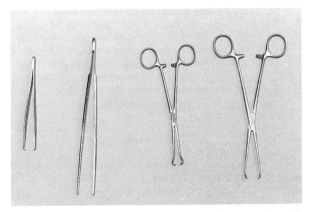

Figure 2–4. Surgical forceps: (*left to right*) Adson, used to pick up skin edges; straight tissue; Allis, used on tougher tissue such as fascia; and Babcock forceps. The Allis and Babcock forceps are sometimes referred to as clamps.

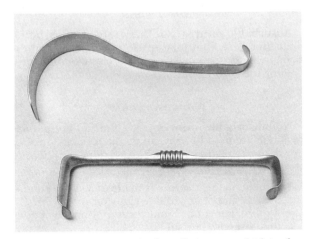

Figure 2–5. (*Top*) Deaver (C-shaped) retractor, which is often used to retract organs (intestine, liver, lung). (*Bottom*) Richardson (L-shaped) body wall retractor.

- The tweezers type is used to pick up skin, fascia, blood vessels, ducts, and organs. These forceps are generally used to pick up the edge of tissues. Examples include Adson's and DeBakey's forceps.

- Hemostat-shaped forceps include the Babcock and the Allis tissue forceps. These instruments ratchet and can be locked in the closed position. They are practical for holding up tissue for long periods of time, thus preventing the finger fatigue that occurs from long grasping with tweezers-type forceps. Babcock forceps are minimally traumatic and are commonly used to hold intestine.

Retractor

The retractor is used to move tissues and organs to gain exposure (see Chapter 1). Retractors may be L-shaped, C-shaped, or shovel-shaped (Fig. 2–5).

SUTURES

Types

Absorbable

Absorbable sutures (e.g., Vicryl) are absorbed by the body over time. They may be used as dermal or subcuticular (under the epidermis) skin closures, thus precluding the need for suture removal (Table 2–2).

Nonabsorbable

Nonabsorbable sutures (e.g., prolene) are permanent and are used in applications such as blood vessel anastomoses or hernia repair where long-term tensile strength is needed, (Table 2–3).

- A monofilament suture is made of a single continuous strand of material (e.g., nylon).
- A multifilament or braided suture is made of multiple strands (e.g., silk).

Sizes

The largest-diameter sutures have a single numerical digit for sizing. The largest (#5) is about the size of string. Zero (0) and #1 are commonly used to close fascia.

Table 2–2. COMMON ABSORBABLE SUTURES

Suture	Material	Duration of Tensile Strength	Common Uses
Chronic catgut	Submucosa of sheep's intestine	5 days	Internal layer gastro-intestinal
Vicryl (Dexon is similar)	Synthetic polygalactic acid (braided)	3 weeks	Internal layer of gastro-intestinal anastomoses Small vessel ligature Subcuticular skin
PDS	Synthetic monofilament polydioxanone	6 weeks	Fascial closure

Table 2–3. COMMON NONABSORBABLE SUTURES

Material	Common Use
Silk-braided	Small-vessel ligature Gut anastomoses
Nylon-monofilament	Skin closure
Prolene-monofilament (polypropylene)	Vascular anastomoses Fascial closure
Braided synthetic polyesters (e.g., mersilene ethibond)	Fascial closure

Smaller sutures are followed by zeros (e.g., 2–0, 3–0, 4–0). The higher the prefix digit, the smaller the suture. Hence, 9–0 and 10–0 are used for ophthalmologic and microvascular work; 3–0 and 4–0 are frequently used on the gastrointestinal tract; 4–0, 5–0, and 6–0 are often used for vascular anastomosis.

3

Orders (Admission, Preop, Postop) and Informed Consent

EVALUATING THE NEWLY ADMITTED PATIENT

No task of the surgical trainee may seem more mundane, yet be more important than the preoperative evaluation. Never skimp on this evaluation. A thorough admitting history and physical may be the only opportunity to find the rectal carcinoma, for example, that would have resulted in disastrous bleeding for the patient while heparinized for cardiac bypass surgery.

PEARL: Call the patients by name and treat them with the utmost respect. No operation is trivial to the person having it. The relationship of surgeon to patient is the most intimate in all of medicine. The patient is turning over complete control to the surgeon. It is your special privilege and responsibility to be the patient's introduction to and guide through the operative experience. Be especially caring and scrupulously honest.

WRITING ORDERS

Each surgeon develops his or her own set of standard guidelines for remembering the preop and postop orders. It is less important which exact mnemonic you use than that you have a system that helps you remember all the important details.

Admission Orders

The following is a sample form used when a patient is admitted:

Admit to (ward)_____ Staff: _____
  Res: _____ Beeper # _____
Diagnosis: _____ Intern: _____
Condition (good/stable/fair/critical):
Vitals: q6h (on routine floor; every hour in ICU [intensive care unit] or intermediate care unit)
Activity: oob (out of bed) ad lib; restrictions (patient-specific)
Allergies: specific or NKDA (no known drug allergies)
Nursing:
  Strict I/O (input and output)
  Preop weight on front of chart
  Daily weights (when indicated)
  ECG (electrocardiogram) (when indicated)
  Chest x-ray (when indicated)
Diet:
  Regular diet (if no comorbid conditions and patient not having bowel surgery)
  Clear liquids (if having bowel surgery)
  NPO (nothing by mouth) after midnight
IV fluids: Determined by patient's condition, for example, start D_5 lactated Ringer's (LR) solution at 100 mL/h 8 hours preop if surgery will be extensive
Meds: Resume all preop meds as appropriate.
  Hold or cut to 50% insulin-sulfonylureas if patient NPO; cover with sliding scale.
Labs: CBC (complete blood count), SMA-6, SMA-12 (Sequential Multiple Analyzer), PT/PTT (prothrombin time-partial thromboplastin time), UA (urinalysis) C&S (culture and sensitivity)

PEARL: In this era of cost containment, the physician should be able to justify every lab test with a specific indication.

Extra: Other x-ray studies, nuclear medicine studies, special procedures, consults, physical therapy, occupational therapy, social services

Consider: DVT (deep venous thrombosis) prophylaxis, sleeping medications

Think of associated illnesses. Patients with chronic renal failure or congestive heart failure should not be fluid-loaded unless your senior team member directs this activity. No routine potassium should be given for renal patients, that is, no lactated Ringer's solution. Insulin management should also be discussed with the senior physician.

Many elective patients have their ECG, chest x-ray, lab tests, and consultations performed in advance. Old charts and the patient's attending physician are the best sources for these records.

Preoperative Note

The preop note is a written checklist in the progress notes confirming that all of the data have been gathered and the patient is ready for surgery. Data to document include the following:

Date: Patient is preop for procedure _____.
CBC:
Chem 7 (electrolyte panel):
PT, PTT
ECG:
Chest x-ray.
Type and screen or type and crossmatch 2, 4, 6 units: specimen in the blood bank.
Consent is on chart.
Preop orders are written.

Preop Orders

Preoperative orders are frequently included in the admission orders.

NPO p (post) midnight
Studies needed:
  Labs

Other studies (e.g., x-rays or pulmonary function tests)
Bowel prep
IV fluids
Preop antibiotics (based on specific indications)

Operative Note

Every patient must have an operative note written in the chart. The operative dictation may take a few days to find the chart, so include the operative findings. Confirm the findings with the primary surgeon.

Preop diagnosis:
Postop diagnosis:
Procedure (list all procedures):
Surgeon (attending):
First assistant (most senior resident):
Second assistant:
Student:
Anesthesia (local, MAC [monitored anesthesia care], epidural, spinal, or GET [general endotracheal tube intubation]):
IV fluids (get from anesthesia):
EBL (estimated blood loss):
Urine output:
Drains (indicate placement):
Specimens:
Complications (be sure to clear this category with the attending):
Findings (if pathology is encountered, diagrams are often useful):
Disposition (to RR in stable condition, extubated):
Date of dictation:

Postop Orders

The following example is for a 53-year-old man who underwent a sigmoid colectomy for colon cancer.

Admit to Ward X Dr. _____ Pager #
_____

Diagnosis: s/p sigmoid colectomy for colon cancer

Condition: stable

Vitals: q2h for 24 hr, then q4h

Call house officer T>38.5°C, P>100 or <60, SBP>160
or <110, RR>30, urine output <60 mL over 2 hrs

Allergies: None

Activity: oob in AM with assistance, ambulate tid (three
times a day)

Nursing:

    Strict I/O, daily weights

    DVT (deep venous thrombosis) prophylaxis: pneu-
matic compression stockings until ambulatory

    Incentive spirometer: 10 puffs q1h while awake

    Drains/tubes: Foley to gravity

        NGT (nasogastric tube) to low constant suction
(sump tube)

        JP (Jackson-Pratt) drain to bulb suction

Diet: NPO

IV fluids: LR @ 125 mL/h for first 24 hours, then change
to maintenance fluid

D_5 1/2 NS or 1/2 NS c̄ 20 mg KCL @ 80 mL/h

Meds: "5 Ps": Preop meds, pain, pee (diuretics), poop,
pus (antibiotics), pillow (sleep, sedation)

    Preop medications: (must be individually reordered)

    Pain regimen: PCA (patient-controlled analgesia) (as
needed)

    Antibiotic: cefotetan 1 g IV q8h if attending wishes to
continue preoperative antibiotics

    Cimetidine: 300 mg IV q8h

AM labs: CBC, SMA-7 (electrolyte panel if indicated)

(Note that postop orders will be patient- and pro-
cedure-specific and that this patient was only one example.)

INFORMED CONSENT

Obtaining the preoperative informed consent is a le-
gal and moral requirement; consent should be obtained
by a physician member of the surgical team. It serves
several purposes:

- Informs the patient of the procedure planned and
ensures that he or she is fully cognizant of the up-
coming events.

- Educates the patient of the risks of the procedure and gives him or her the opportunity to ask further questions.
- Acts as the admission ticket to the operating room.

PEARL: Obtain informed consent as early in the day as possible. Adequate time should be allowed to answer the patient's questions. Demonstrating the probable location of the incision site and discussing postoperative tubes and IV lines and any potential for ICU admission will help allay the patient's fear and anxiety. Pain and pain management should be discussed, as well as any preoperative arrangements for and intraoperative risks of blood transfusions. For patients having elective surgery, generally the attending has discussed the procedure in detail. The role of the written preop consent form is confirmation and documentation.

A senior resident or attending physician will discuss the procedure with the patient. This discussion should include the following:

- Outline of the indications for operation.
- List of the essential features of the procedure.
- Discussion of the intraoperative and postoperative risks and any expected changes in normal activities after recovery.

Summarize the informed consent discussion on the hospital chart, and document the reasons for and goals of the operation, the expected benefit, and the risks. The resident should state that in his or her judgment the patient and family understood and accepted the operative recommendation. This documentation is of critical medicolegal importance.

4
CHAPTER

Fluids and Electrolytes

The subject of fluids and electrolytes often evokes confusion for medical students and residents. This chapter presents one approach to fluid and electrolyte therapy in surgical practice, and provides the basis for answering two questions:

- Which intravenous solutions should be given?
- How much fluid should be given to surgical patients?

FLUID COMPARTMENTS

Figure 4–1 depicts the common fluid compartments in the human body, their relationship to total body water and body weight, and their average volumes. **PEARL: Total body water (TBW) is 60% of body weight, with two thirds being intracellular fluid (ICF) and one third being extracellular fluid (ECF).**

ICF, the larger of the two compartments, equals 40% of body weight. This fluid is found inside cells, mostly in muscle. ECF equals 20% of body weight and represents fluid not located within cells. It is the more clinically relevant compartment and is composed of interstitial (extravascular, extracellular) fluid and plasma. Interstitial fluid is three-fourths of ECF or 15% of body weight, and plasma volume is one-fourth of ECF or 5%

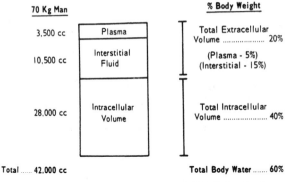

Figure 4–1. Functional compartments of body fluids. (From Shires GT, Canizaro PC: Fluid and electrolyte management of the surgical patient. In Sabiston DC Jr, [ed]. Textbook of Surgery, 13th ed. Philadelphia, WB Saunders, 1986:64.)

of body weight. As clinicians, we interact with the plasma volume, but it is important to appreciate that this compartment represents the "tip of the iceberg" of TBW. This is why so much potassium (K^+) must be administered to correct hypokalemia. For example, with a serum K^+ of 3.0, you can calculate how much K^+ is needed to restore the level to 4.0 in the 3.5-liter plasma volume. Plasma volume, however, is in equilibrium with the 10.5-liter interstitial fluid compartment and it too must have its K^+ level increased.

Another important fluid volume to consider is total blood volume. **PEARL: Total blood volume is 7% of body weight or, on average, 5 liters in an adult.** This is important to know in order to estimate percent of blood loss and categorize the severity of hemorrhagic shock (see "Hypovolemic and Hemorrhagic Shock" in Chapter 24).

Electrolyte Composition of Fluid Compartments

Figure 4–2 depicts the anion and cation content of the three major fluid compartments and presents some important values and relationships that you should be familiar with.

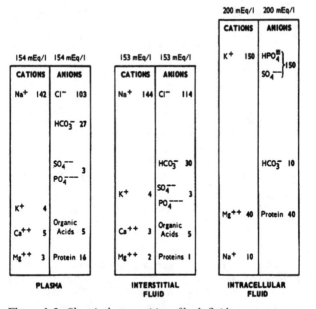

Figure 4–2. Chemical composition of body fluid compartments. (From Shires GT, Canizaro PC: Fluid and electrolyte management of the surgical patient. In Sabiston DC Jr, [ed]. Textbook of Surgery, 13th ed. Philadelphia, WB Saunders, 1986:65.)

Plasma volume contains 154 mEq per liter of cations and 154 mEq per liter of anions. (These details are important because an IV fluid was developed to exactly match them, as you'll see later.) The specific composition resembles a routine serum electrolyte panel. The major cation is Na^+, and the minor cations are K^+, Ca^{2+}, and Mg^{2+}. The predominant anions are Cl^- and HCO_3^- (bicarbonate). A modest anion contribution from plasma proteins is derived from the negative charges associated with some amino acids.

Interstitial fluid is separated from plasma by the passive highly permeable capillary endothelial barrier. This allows easy passage of small electrolytes and limited passage of large macromolecules (proteins). Therefore, it is easy to predict the composition of this fluid compartment.

The cation composition is essentially the same as plasma. The anion composition differs because the contribution of proteins drops to 1 mEq per liter, and the difference is made up by an increase in Cl^- and HCO_3^-.

ICF is separated from interstitial fluid by the active, essentially nonpermeable, cell membrane. One of the cell membrane's important functions is to actively pump Na^+ out and K^+ in via the energy-dependent $Na^+ K^+$ adenosine triphosphatase (ATPase) pump. This accounts for the near reversal in Na^+ and K^+ content within cells. The major intracellular cations are K^+ at 150 mEq per liter, and Na^+ is diminished to 10 mEq per liter. Sulfates and phosphates are the predominant intracellular anions, with a significant contribution from protein.

Normal Fluid and Solute Balance

Table 4–1 shows average water "ins and outs" for a 70-kg adult. With our intake of oral fluids and solids, we put out about 800 to 1500 mL of urine and up to 250 mL of water in stool daily.

We take in about 100 mEq per day of Na^+ and 50 mEq per day of K^+. Losses through urine, sweat, and intestines balance this gain.

Volume and Composition of Gastrointestinal Secretions

The volume and composition of various gastrointestinal (GI) secretions are listed in Table 4–2. Many surgical patients suffer depletion of one or more of these fluids, therefore several principles from this table should be remembered.

1. **PEARL: The deeper into the GI tract, the more plasma-like are the secretions in their composition.**
2. Secretions made in any GI tract segment or organ are normally absorbed in more distal portions of the GI tract (e.g., the small bowel) and hence contribute to overall fluid, electrolyte, and acid-base balance.
3. Each organ has one or two outstanding electrolyte compositions that are noteworthy.

Table 4–1. WATER INTAKE AND OUTPUT

H$_2$O Gain—Routes	Average Daily Volume (mL)
Sensible	
Oral fluids	800–1500
Solid foods	500–700
H$_2$O Loss—Routes	
Sensible	
Urine	800–1600
Intestinal	0–250
Sweat	0
Insensible	
Lungs and skin	600–900

Adapted from Shires GT, Canizaro PC: Fluid and electrolyte management of the surgical patient. In Sabiston DC Jr, (ed). Textbook of Surgery, 13th ed. Philadelphia, WB Saunders, 1986:77.

Table 4–2. COMPOSITION OF GASTROINTESTINAL SECRETIONS

	Volume (mL/24 hr)	Na$^+$ (mEq/L)	K$^+$ (mEq/L)	Cl$^-$ (mEq/L)	HCO$_3^-$ (mEq/L)
Salivary	1500	10	26	10	30
Stomach	1500	60	10	130	—
Duodenum	1000	140	5	80	—
Ileum	3000	140	5	104	30
Colon	—	60	30	40	—
Pancreas	500	140	5	75	115
Bile	500	145	5	100	35

Adapted from Shires GT, Canizaro PC: Fluid and electrolyte management of the surgical patient. In Sabiston DC Jr, (ed). Textbook of Surgery, 13th ed. Philadelphia, WB Saunders, 1986:74.

Salivary Secretions

Salivary secretions amount to about 1500 mL per day. We swallow all our saliva and only appreciate this volume in patients who cannot swallow their salivary secretions (e.g., esophageal obstruction due to cancer, after severe strokes and after major head and neck surgery). Saliva is relatively low in electrolytes, but notable for high K^+ and HCO_3^- content.

Gastric Secretions

Gastric secretions are lost in many of our patients via nasogastric (NG) tubes on suction. **PEARL: The stomach secretes about 1500 mL per day of a fluid rich in K^+, Cl^-, and H^+.** Therefore, a patient with an NG tube or a gastric outlet obstruction (with vomiting), if untreated, will develop severe dehydration and a hypokalemic, hypochloremic metabolic alkalosis.

Secretions of the Ileum

The ileum, mainly thought of as an absorptive organ, secretes about 3000 mL per day of a plasma-like fluid. This fluid is normally absorbed by the small bowel and colon. Any condition that causes the accumulation of these secretions in the bowel and impairs subsequent absorption can cause rapid and severe dehydration and electrolyte depletion. We see these problems in patients with mechanical small-bowel obstruction and paralytic ileus (nonfunctioning of the bowels) due to intra-abdominal infections or ileus after major intra-abdominal operations. In these situations, small bowel secretions build up in the intestines, are not completely absorbed, and therefore cannot contribute to overall fluid and electrolyte balance. Aggressive fluid and electrolyte replacement therapy with a plasma-like fluid (i.e., lactated Ringer's solution) is indicated. **PEARL: Small bowel fluid is plasma-like in composition, and, when it is not being absorbed (e.g., ileus, small bowel obstruction, intra-abdominal inflammation), a plasma-like fluid deficit develops.**

Pancreatic and Bile Secretions

The pancreas secretes about 500 mL per day of a fluid that is very plasma-like except for very high HCO_3^- (115 mEq/L). Therefore, in patients whose pancreatic secretions do not enter the GI tract for subsequent absorption (e.g., pancreaticocutaneous fistula as a complication of pancreatic surgery, trauma, or pancreatitis), IV fluids need to be supplemented with HCO_3^- to prevent a metabolic acidosis from developing.

Bile secretions account for about 500 mL per day and are plasma-like except for a slightly elevated HCO_3^- concentration (35 mEq/L). A patient who undergoes a common bile duct exploration and has a T-tube draining the common bile duct for a week or so postoperatively is likely to develop a metabolic acidosis unless HCO_3^- supplementation is given.

IV SOLUTIONS

Table 4–3 lists the types and electrolyte composition of common IV solutions. You need to determine the exact composition of two of these fluids. By doing so, you will be able to figure out the composition of all of them. **PEARL: The two key fluids to commit to memory are normal saline (NS) and lactated Ringer's (LR) solution. NS contains 154 mEq/L of Na^+ and Cl^-. LR contains 130 mEq/L of Na^+, 109 of Cl^-, 28 of lactate, and 3 of Ca^{2+}.**

IV fluids are divided into two major categories: crystalloid and colloid.

- Crystalloid solutions are clear, transparent solutions of electrolytes and dextrose. **PEARL: Crystalloid solutions are the most important and widely used category of fluid.**
- Colloid solutions may or may not be clear. They contain macromolecules (either proteins or starches) that give the solution oncotic force.

Crystalloids

Normal Saline Solutions

The classic crystalloid solution is NS or 0.9% sodium chloride (NaCl). It contains 154 mEq/L of Na^+ and 154 mEq/L of Cl^-. These numbers reflect the total cation and anion content of plasma, and NS is designed to match that total with the two predominant electrolytes. NS is an isotonic solution because its tonicity or osmolality closely matches that of plasma—around 300 mOsm/L.

Table 4–3. ELECTROLYTE COMPOSITION OF COMMERCIALLY AVAILABLE INTRAVENOUS SOLUTIONS

	Na^+	Cl^-	K^+	HCO_3^-	Ca^{2+}	Osm	Calories/liter
Crystalloid							
0.9% NaCl (NS)	154	154				292	
0.9% NaCl + 5% dextrose (D_5 NS)	154	154				565	200
0.45% NaCl (½ NS)	77	77				146	
0.45% NaCl + 5% dextrose (D_5 ½ NS)	77	77				420	200
0.2% NaCl + 5% dextrose (D_5 ¼ NS)	34	34				330	200
5% dextrose in water (D_5W)						274	200
10% dextrose in water (D_{10}W)						548	400
Lactated Ringer's (LR)	130	109	4	28*	3	277	
3% NaCl	513	513				960	
Colloid							
HESPAN	154	154				310	
5% plasma protein factor (plasminate)	145	100	0.25				
25% albumin	130–160	130–160	1				

*Present in solution as lactate, which is metabolized to HCO_3^-.
Adapted from Taylor DS: Fluid and electrolytes. In Lyerly HK, (ed). The Handbook of Surgical Intensive Care, 2nd ed. Chicago, Year Book Medical Publishers, 1989:230.

D_5NS is normal saline with 5% dextrose or 50 g dextrose per liter. The dextrose increases the osmolality of the solution to 565 mOsm/L, but this is safe because it is rapidly diluted in the plasma and interstitial volume. The dextrose provides 200 calories of carbohydrate (carbohydrate provides 4 Kcal/g). **PEARL: Dextrose 5% is added to IV solutions for its protein-sparing effect in the fasting patient.** The reason for adding 5% dextrose to IV solutions, particularly for patients who are fasting, is to stimulate the body into releasing insulin, the major anabolic hormone, which spares protein stores from gluconeogenesis for up to 10 to 14 days in the fasting state.

Half NS has half the Na^+ and Cl^- content of NS. It is a hypotonic solution because its osmolality is significantly less than that of plasma. It is available with or without 5% dextrose. Quarter NS has only 34 mEq/L of both Na^+ and Cl^-, and, owing to the dangerous hypotonicity that such a solution presents, it is only provided with 5% dextrose to raise its osmolality to a safe level. D_5W is rarely used in surgical patients. It is occasionally needed to avoid any salt in postoperative cirrhotic patients (who avidly retain any given salt and thus water, often in the form of ascites) or in patients who have large free water deficits that require correction.

Lactated Ringer's Solution

LR is the preferred isotonic crystalloid solution of surgeons because it most closely resembles the composition of plasma (and interstitial fluid) and because many surgical patients need restoration of intravascular and interstitial fluid. Its composition is listed in Table 4–3. **PEARL: The lactate in LR is rapidly metabolized to HCO_3^- by the liver, then converted to CO_2 in the blood and blown off by the lungs. It rarely affects pH.** (Isolyte is a preferred isotonic crystalloid solution of anesthetists for intraoperative use and is very similar to LR.)

Colloids

The classic colloid solution is plasminate, an electrolyte solution containing 5% plasma proteins. The most commonly used colloid solution today is Hespan, an NS-based solution containing a complex starch macromolecule for its oncotic force. Although these solutions remain in the intravascular space in the short run (hours), they eventually leak out of the intravascular space (within 12 to 24 hours).

In surgery, use of colloids is limited. One use, however, is in patients undergoing open heart surgery on cardiopulmonary bypass. Colloids have a role in increasing preload to improve cardiac function as the patient comes off bypass, but avoiding the larger volumes of crystalloid that would otherwise be required.

PRACTICAL FLUID AND ELECTROLYTE THERAPY IN SURGICAL PATIENTS

Selecting an IV Solution

PEARL: When selecting an appropriate IV solution for a patient, decide whether the patient requires maintenance fluids or resuscitation fluids.

- Maintenance fluids are required for patients who are not stressed but are NPO (nothing by mouth) and are not having any GI secretions removed from their bodies.
- Resuscitation fluids are required for patients who have had or are having ongoing fluid losses either in the form of blood (e.g., gunshot wound to chest with massive hemothorax) or extracellular fluid (e.g., gastric outlet obstruction with vomiting, intra-abdominal sepsis with ileus, continuous NG suction).

PEARL: On surgical service, it is better to err on the side of additional resuscitation in borderline cases (e.g., the postoperative patient with an NG tube inserted or the patient with an ileus who is not absorbing plasma-like ileal secretions).

If the patient requires maintenance fluids only, an appropriate choice would be a hypotonic crystalloid solution with some added K^+ tailored to meet total daily fluid (2000 to 2500 mL) and electrolyte (Na^+, 100 mEq; K^+, 50 mEq) requirements. In fact, the best fluid to accomplish this is $D_5\frac{1}{4}NS$ with 10 to 20 mEq/L KCl. At a maintenance rate of 100 mL/hour, this provides

2400 mL of fluid, 82 mEq of Na^+, and 24 to 48 mEq of K^+. Although ½NS would be tolerated by most healthy patients, the extra Na^+ load (185 mEq) it provides is nearly double the requirement. An older patient population, however, often has medical problems such as congestive heart failure or renal insufficiency. For them, this extra salt load may be hazardous and is therefore not warranted for maintenance fluid and electrolyte requirements.

PEARL: If a patient requires resuscitation, the only appropriate IV solution choice is isotonic crystalloid. The only two choices in this category are LR or NS. In most cases, the NS and LR are interchangeable. Surgeons favor LR, but NS accomplishes the same goal. If one is not available, ask for the other without hesitation. **PEARL: Dextrose is avoided for aggressive resuscitation because the body utilizes dextrose poorly in settings of severe stress, thus resulting in hyperglycemia. Hyperglycemia can cause an osmotic diuresis that will complicate the use of urine output as an accurate monitor of resuscitation.** (Dextrose should be added after aggressive resuscitation is completed in 1 to 2 days). In these severe settings, an initial 1- to 2-L bolus of fluid should be given over ½ to 2 hours and then fluids should be run at a rate of at least 150 mL per hour (and often at a much higher rate).

PEARL: A common error is to run resuscitation fluids at only 125 or 150 mL per hour without a bolus. This is much too slow for the needs of a seriously ill patient and for any surgeon's comfort level. Volume deficits must be restored rapidly in such clinical settings to avoid adverse complications.

COMMON CLINICAL SCENARIOS

Gastric Outlet Obstruction

Patients suffering from gastric outlet obstruction who are unable to eat and have continued vomiting present with profound dehydration and a hypokalemic, hypochloremic metabolic alkalosis. This is due to the loss of gastric secretions (high in K^+, Cl^-, and H^+). In this setting, follow these guidelines:

- Isotonic crystalloid resuscitation should begin with a fluid that does not contain K^+ because adminis-

tering K^+ can lead to hyperkalemia if acute renal failure has set in.
- NS should initially be used to treat the intravascular depletion.
- The electrolyte and acid-base disturbances often correct on their own after resuscitation. If they do not correct, specific K^+ replacement should be given after intravascular volume has been restored and urine output established.

Open Intra-abdominal Surgery

PEARL: During surgery with an open peritoneal cavity, fluid requirements are about 1000 mL/hr, mostly because of a 10 mL/kg/hr evaporative fluid loss. The addition of 100 mL per hour for maintenance requirements, some blood loss and fluid sequestration in surgically injured tissues, and ileus results in a total resuscitative fluid requirement of about 1000 mL per hour.

During surgery, patients receive large volumes of isotonic, crystalloid fluids. The evaporative losses stop after the abdomen is closed. Third-space losses above maintenance requirements continue, however, because of the postoperative ileus, which allows accumulation of plasma-like ileal fluid within the bowel, edema within the bowel wall, and edema in the surgical area of injury. An NG tube is often in place removing additional fluids. For these reasons, continued resuscitation with an isotonic, crystalloid fluid is required postoperatively.

We recommend LR at about 150 mL/hour for most adult patients. These increased fluid requirements continue for about 24 to 48 hours. When the normal postoperative diuretic phase begins and the additional fluid is mobilized and diuresed, IV fluids can be changed to maintenance requirements or slightly less.

Nasogastric Tube

For patients with an NG tube, administration of a maintenance IV of D_5 ¼ NS with 10 mEq/L KCl at 80 to 100 mL per hour and replacement of NG losses milliliter per milliliter per shift with LR and 20 mEq/L KCl

Table 4-4. COMMON ELECTROLYTE DISORDERS

Electrolyte Disorder	Etiology	Signs and Symptoms	Treatment
Hyperkalemia	Renal insufficiency, acidosis, tissue necrosis (hemolysis in specimen)	Weakness, loss of deep tendon reflexes, diarrhea, ECG changes (peaked T waves)	Saline hydration, diuretic therapy, Kayexalate, insulin, and D_{50} if severe
Hypokalemia	Renal losses (diuretics), vomiting or NG suction, alkalosis	Weakness, ileus, ECG changes (flattened T waves)	Oral and IV potassium
Hypernatremia	Dehydration, diabetes insipidus	Mental status changes, thirst, seizures	Provide free water (D_5W)
Hyponatremia	Dilutional (too much free water), syndrome of inappropriate antidiuretic hormone secretion	Confusion, lethargy, seizures	Correct underlying disorder, water restriction, 3% NaCl if seizures
Hypercalcemia	Hyperparathyroidism, malignancy	Polyuria, mental status changes, abdominal pain	Saline hydration, diuretic therapy, diphosphanates
Hypocalcemia	Hypoalbuminemia, hypoparathyroidism, alkalosis	Numbness, paresthesias	Oral and IV calcium, vitamin D

is the most accurate method. Running two IV lines is cumbersome, so we usually combine the fluid requirements into a single IV and run D_5 ½ NS with 20 mEq/L KCl at 125 mL/hour. This satisfies both maintenance needs and the additional resuscitative requirements.

Specific Electrolyte Disorders

Detailed reviews of each type of electrolyte disorder are beyond the scope of this handbook. Table 4–4 summarizes the common electrolyte disorders.

5
CHAPTER

Principles of Surgical Oncology

GENERAL CONSIDERATIONS

A diagnosis of cancer strikes fear in the minds of the patient and family members. Therefore, the clinician must not only address the cancer but also help other health care providers in caring for the emotional needs of the patient and family. When discussing malignancies with patients and families, keep the following in mind:

- *Patients commonly react in a way to signal when they have heard enough.* A discussion of a "lump," "mass," "tumor," or "lesion" can lead up to the words "cancer" or "malignancy." Patients who break down in tears should be given time to compose themselves.
- *Patients and families frequently forget what they have been told at the first meeting with the physician.* You may have to repeat the information at a subsequent time.

Physicians have four weapons against cancers: surgery, chemotherapy, radiation therapy, and, in some cases, immunotherapy. Cancers are most frequently cared for with an interdisciplinary team approach. In most centers, a weekly tumor board conference is held and attended by oncologists, surgeons, radiotherapists, and pathologists. There cancer cases are discussed in detail, and a plan for care is recommended.

Surgeons become involved with cancer cases for a variety of reasons, including establishing a diagnosis (frequently by biopsy), resecting for cure, operating for palliation, and occasionally operating for "debulking." Some tumors, such as thyroid cancer, are readily cured by surgery; others, such as pancreatic cancer, are not.

ESTABLISHING A DIAGNOSIS

PEARL: The least invasive means of obtaining tissue from a tumor is by fine-needle aspiration (FNA) for cytology. The cell samples obtained are processed and evaluated like the Pap smear. For most tumors, FNA has sensitivities and specificities of 80 to 90%.

The following are other methods of obtaining tissue:

- **Needle biopsy** with a larger-bore device (e.g., "true-cut") obtains a core of tissue for histologic examination.
- **Incisional biopsy** involves removing a portion of a tumor for histologic examination; it is usually used for large bulky tumors.
- **Excisional biopsy** involves removing the entire tumor for histologic examination; it is frequently used for small tumors.

RESECTING FOR CURE

During surgery for cure of a cancer, two main principles are followed:

- The surgeon attempts to resect the organ or organ segment containing the tumor with "clear margins." This means that on histologic examination no cancer cells are visible at any margin of the resected specimen.
- Most cancer surgery involves enbloc resection of the organ (or organ segment) plus the lymphatic drainage of that organ or organ segment.

CONTROVERSY: It is not known whether radical lymph node dissection actually increases cure rates or simply offers better staging.

Perhaps the best illustration of this controversy is breast cancer. During the 1960s, surgeons developed increasingly radical operations for breast cancer. The belief was that the cancer advanced locally and via local lymphatics millimeter by millimeter. Therefore, resecting more and more tissue locally (such as the chest wall) and more lymph nodes would increase survival rates. This concept failed to prove true. During the 1980s, most clinicians and investigators believed that lymph node involvement with metastatic breast cancer cells indicated not just local spread but systemic disease. This improved understanding of cancer biology led to changes in therapy, as outlined in Chapter 8.

The failure of the theory that more and more radical resections should be done in cancer surgery is especially true for cancers of the GI tract and breast and in melanoma. Nevertheless, radical resection has *limited success* in the following:

1. Head and neck cancer (frequently being supplanted by multimodality treatment).
2. Tumors unresponsive to chemotherapy and resistant to radiation therapy, such as thyroid cancers and soft tissue sarcomas (Surgery represents the only hope for cure.)

In fact, the cure rate for thyroid cancer with surgical therapy is very high (see Chapter 9).

OPERATING FOR PALLIATION

Palliative surgery involves resecting a tumor in a situation in which a surgical cure is not possible. The most common indications for palliative surgery are

- To relieve pain
- To stop bleeding
- To alleviate obstruction of the GI tract

Palliative surgery is frequently required for noncurable tumors of the GI tract. Examples would be gastric or colonic tumors that are bleeding but cannot be cured owing to widespread metastases.

DEBULKING

Debulking (cytoreductive surgery) involves removing large portions of tumors to increase the chances of survival with subsequent other cancer therapies.

PEARL: The concept of debulking a tumor is invalid for most tumors.

Debulking does, however, have a role in patients with the following cancers:

- **Ovarian and testicular carcinoma.** Patients' survival is improved with subsequent chemotherapy and radiation therapy after debulking. In these situations, the residual tumor load visible to the naked eye should be 1 cm^2 or less.
- **Noncurable endocrine tumors.** Patients with tumors such as metastatic pheochromocytoma and insulinoma may have a clinical syndrome caused by excess hormone secretion by the tumor. These are patients for whom medical therapy no longer controls the symptoms of the disease. In some cases, debulking lowers hormone concentrations to subclinical levels.

6
CHAPTER

Principles of Transplantation

TRANSPLANT IMMUNOLOGY

The Rejection Response

Transplant rejection occurs when the donor organ is recognized as **foreign** by the host. Such recognition involves identification and comparison of certain protein and glycoprotein antigens, chiefly those of the major histocompatibility complex (MHC), referred to as the human leukocyte antigen (HLA) complex. Genes coding for these antigens are found on chromosome 6.

Class I MHC antigens are found on a variety of cell types and are the targets for cytolytic T cells. Class II antigens are found on lymphocytes and are recognized by helper T cells. Tissue typing and crossmatching involve identification of class I (A and B loci) and class II MHC antigens. Table 6–1 is an example of the crossmatching used in transplantation.

Antigen-presenting cells (APCs) take up donor antigen and reexpress donor class II antigen on their surface in conjunction with host class II antigen. Comparisons between "self" and "non-self" (foreign cells) are then made by the immune system, and non-self pairings stimulate a response.

Lymphocyte populations can be identified by a variety of surface markers (e.g., CD3, CD4, CD8). Helper T

**Table 6–1. CROSSMATCHING USED
IN TRANSPLANTATION**

Organ	ABO	HLA	Cytotoxic
Kidney	+	+	+
Liver	+	+	−*
Pancreas	+	+	+
Lung	+		−
Heart	+		+†

*Unknown whether classic hyperacute rejection definitely occurs.
†Not done for every case.

cells are CD4-positive (CD4+). They use CD4 in combination with the CD3 receptor and other adhesion molecules to bind to the APC. Helper T cells then become activated and produce interleukin-2 (IL-2) and other lymphokines. IL-2 further stimulates helper T-cell activation and clonal expansion and activates cytotoxic T cells. These cytotoxic cells are CD8+ and use this receptor to bind the foreign class I antigen after they have migrated into the transplanted organ. Once bound, the CD8+ T cells induce target cell lysis. **PEARL: Class II antigens stimulate helper T cells and class I T cells preferentially.** In addition to the cell-mediated immune response, donor antigen can elicit a humoral response by stimulating helper T cells to induce antibody production by B lymphocytes.

Three types of rejection are classically described:

1. **Hyperacute rejection** occurs within minutes of donor organ reperfusion and is antibody- and complement-mediated. The transplant becomes dusky and edematous while still in the operating room. No effective treatment is known except for graft excision. In hyperacute rejection, the responsible cytotoxic antibodies are present in the recipient before the transplant is introduced. This is well described in the literature for renal transplantation but is not well described for other organ transplantations.

2. **Acute rejection** occurs days to months after transplantation and involves the cellular immune response described above.

3. **Chronic rejection** takes place months to years after transplantation and involves both cellular and humoral immune responses.

IMMUNOSUPPRESSION

PEARL: Immunosuppression is the cornerstone of postoperative management of the transplant patient. The goal of immunosuppression in transplantation is to achieve selective blockade of the immune response (to prevent graft rejection) without causing severe generalized impairment of immunity that would lead to frequent and possibly life-threatening infections.

Most protocols involve corticosteroids and one or two additional agents, as shown in Table 6–2.

KIDNEY TRANSPLANTATION

Renal transplantation is indicated for patients with end-stage renal disease.

PEARL: Contraindications to kidney transplantation include cancer, infection, and advanced age.

Transplants are typically in the right iliac fossa with vascular anastomoses to the right external or common iliac artery and right common iliac vein. The ureter is anastomosed to the bladder using a submuscular tunnel to prevent reflux.

Most patients with renal transplants experience at least one episode of acute rejection. However, 50% of cadaveric grafts remain functional at 10 years, and more than 75% of living related transplants function a decade after implantation.

Frequent episodes of acute rejection are associated with the development of chronic rejection. *Chronic rejection* is evident as a steady decline in renal function and rise in serum creatinine levels after transplantation. Recurrence of the underlying disease may also be responsible for late graft loss.

PEARL: Rejection must be differentiated from vascular and urologic problems. This is particularly true early after transplantation.

Such differentiation is accomplished with a renal scan, which assesses both renal blood flow and function.

Table 6–2. IMMUNOSUPPRESSIVE AGENTS

Agent	Mechanism of Action	Side Effect
Cyclosporine	Inhibits T-cell activation	Nephrotoxicity, tremors, hypertension, gingival hyperplasia
FK506 (Tacrolimus)	Inhibits T-cell activation	Less nephrotoxic than cyclosporine
Azathioprine	Inhibits purine synthesis (after conversion of 6-MP)	Leukopenia
Antilymphocytic globulin	Polyclonal serum to human lymphocytes promotes clearance of lymphocytes	Chills, fever, rash, leukopenia
OKT₃ (monoclonal antibody to T-cells)	Monoclonal antibody to CD3 complex, depletes functioning T cells	Fever, pulmonary edema
Corticosteroids	↓Neutrophil migration and enzyme release ↓Effective antigen presentation ↓Cytokine production (IFN-γ) ↓Acute inflammatory mediators and vascular permeability	Diabetes, hypertension, cataracts, Cushing's syndrome

IFN = interferon; IL = interleukin; MP = mercaptopurine.

Occasionally, a percutaneous biopsy is needed to definitively demonstrate histologic evidence of rejection. Possible vascular and urologic problems that must be differentiated from transplant rejection are lymphoceles in the graft pocket, which can cause painful swelling of both the graft area and the ipsilateral lower extremity, and fluid collections, which can compress the vascular supply or ureter.

PANCREAS TRANSPLANTATION

Pancreas transplantation is indicated for type I diabetes in selected patients. In patients with diabetic nephropathy, pancreas transplantation may be performed in concert with a renal transplantation.

The following are considerations for pancreas transplantation:

- Allograft exocrine secretions may be handled by ductal obstruction with direct ductal instillation of sclerosants, anastomosis to the small bowel, or anastomosis to the bladder.
- Endocrine function is typically well preserved.

Most patients discontinue exogenous insulin and experience fewer chronic diabetes-related complications. Of all pancreas transplants, 75% remain functional at one year.

LIVER TRANSPLANTATION

Liver transplantation is indicated for patients with the following conditions:

- End-stage liver disease secondary to chronic active hepatitis (most common)
- Alcoholic liver disease
- Primary biliary cirrhosis
- Sclerosing cholangitis
- Biliary atresia in children

Patients who are active on transplant lists commonly have experienced complications of liver disease (variceal bleeding, encephalopathy, ascites) or laboratory evidence of significantly impaired hepatic function (e.g., bilirubin >5, albumin <2.5, prolonged prothrombin time [PT]).

Operations are typically done on vena caval bypass without systemic heparinization (heparin-coated circuits only). Implantation is orthotopic and involves a biliary anastomosis to the recipient bile duct or jejunum. Rejection is commonly treated with steroids and OKT_3 (a monoclonal antibody to T-cells) or FK506 (tacrolimus, an immunosuppressive drug).

A year after transplantation 75% of liver allografts remain functional.

CARDIAC TRANSPLANTATION

Heart transplantation is indicated for patients with end-stage cardiac disease (without fixed pulmonary hypertension).

The following are *contraindications* for cardiac transplantation:

- Irreversible liver, kidney, central nervous system (CNS), or pulmonary dysfunction
- Cancer
- Active infection
- Age over 60 or 65 years (at most centers)
- Peripheral vascular disease (relative contraindication)

Transplantation is orthotopic with left atrial-atrial anastomosis followed by right atrial-atrial or bicaval anastomoses. The aorta is subsequently anastomosed distal to the coronary ostia, the cross clamp is removed, and the pulmonary artery is connected.

The right ventricle is most prone to reversible dysfunction early after transplantation, and, accordingly, volume overload is avoided. Diastolic filling time is kept short by maintaining the heart rate of approximately 110 to 120 using pharmaceutical agents such as isoproterenol (Isuprel). Pulmonary vascular resistance is similarly minimized.

Rejection

Rejection is monitored with scheduled transvenous endomyocardial biopsies. Infection remains a significant cause of morbidity, and chronic rejection is evident as graft atherosclerosis (often missed with left heart catheterization).

The one-year survival rate is nearly 90%.

LUNG TRANSPLANTATION

Types

Single-lung transplantation is indicated for severe emphysema, pulmonary fibrosis, or sarcoid.

Double-lung transplantation is required for septic lung disease (bronchiectasis, cystic fibrosis) to avoid infection from a remaining native lung.

Pulmonary hypertension can be treated with single- or double-lung transplantation. Some authorities believe that pulmonary hypertension is more likely to recur in patients given only a single lung. Heart-lung transplantation is indicated for severe pulmonary disease with associated irreversible cardiac dysfunction (end stage pulmonary hypertension).

Morbidity and Mortality

Causes of morbidity include infection (especially cytomegalovirus [CMV]) and rejection. Rejection episodes occur more often early after surgery but gradually become less frequent with time. Unfortunately, numerous episodes of acute rejection correlate with the development of obliterative bronchiolitis later on.

PEARL: Obliterative bronchiolitis is a manifestation of chronic rejection, is poorly understood, and has little effective therapy.

Obliterative bronchiolitis is typically progressive and is marked by increasing dyspnea and declining pulmonary function.

Nearly 70% of single-lung transplant recipients, but fewer than 60% of heart-lung recipients, are alive one year after transplantation.

7
CHAPTER

Minimally Invasive Surgery

GENERAL BACKGROUND

Until the advent of anesthesia in the late nineteenth century, surgery was limited by the pain inflicted. General anesthesia greatly expanded the success of surgical therapy, but patients remained apprehensive about postoperative pain. Imaging, fiber optics, and computer technology led to the concept of minimally invasive surgery, or "band aid" surgery. These procedures can be performed through cylindrical trocars, or ports, which are placed through 0.5- to 2-cm incisions or stab wounds. Telescopic cameras and instruments are placed through the ports, and the surgeon works while watching the procedure on a television monitor. At the end of the procedure, the trocars are removed, and the trocar incisions are closed.

Endoscopy, arthroscopy, and cystoscopy have evolved from being purely diagnostic to becoming more therapeutic, based on laparoscopic technology and refinements in instrumentation.

PEARL: The major advantage of minimally invasive surgery is less post-procedure pain. Pain is a major trigger to the neuroendocrine stress response to surgery.

The following are advantages of minimally invasive surgery:

- Major fluid shifts are less common.
- Prolonged postop ileus is less common.
- The patient is ambulatory sooner, has less pain, and may anticipate an earlier return to normal activity levels.

LAPAROSCOPY

Laparoscopy is telescopic examination within the peritoneal cavity. It began as a diagnostic tool for the gynecologist. Now many intra-abdominal procedures can be performed under laparoscopic conditions (Table 7–1). The procedure is as follows. (Note that patients with prior abdominal surgery may have adhesions. In these patients, the needle insufflation is omitted, and the first trocar is placed by direct fascial cut down.)

- A needle is placed in the peritoneum via a small periumbilical incision.
- The peritoneal cavity is then filled with CO_2 to a pressure of 15 mm Hg (inflating the peritoneal cavity like a balloon). This requires 4 to 5 liters of CO_2.
- With the cavity inflated, a telescopic camera is placed, and the surgeon can view intra-abdominal organs on the screen.

Laparoscopic Cholecystectomy

The first general surgical operation developed using laparoscopic techniques was cholecystectomy. Laparoscopic cholecystectomy proceeds as follows:

Table 7–1. LAPAROSCOPIC PROCEDURES

Common	Less Common
Cholecystectomy	Splenectomy
Appendectomy	Peptic ulcer surgery
Hernia repair	Adrenalectomy
Antireflux surgery (fundoplication)	
Colectomy	

- The gallbladder is grasped with an instrument and retracted cephalad over the superior surface of the liver. This allows excellent visualization of the **triangle of Calot,** an anatomic triangle defined by the liver edge, the common bile duct, and the cystic duct.
- The cystic duct and cystic artery are divided between metallic clips.
- The gallbladder is then dissected from the hepatic bed using electrocautery or, less commonly, laser.
- Once free, the gallbladder is removed via a trocar site and sent to pathology.

Laparoscopic cholecystectomy has changed biliary surgery.

PEARL: A major advantage of laparoscopic cholecystectomy is a reduced hospital stay. Generally, patients having a laparoscopic cholecystectomy go home the same day or on the first postop day. Open cholecystectomy frequently requires a 3- to 5-day hospital stay.

Most cholecystectomies in the United States are now done laparoscopically. A disadvantage of laparoscopic cholecystectomy is an increase in common bile duct injury (compared with "open" biliary surgery). The incidence of bile duct injury in open cholecystectomy is 1 to 2 per 1000 operations. In laparoscopic cholecystectomy, the bile duct injury rate is about five times as great. This is a serious complication that extends operation time or requires additional operations.

Inguinal Hernia Repair

Inguinal hernia repair performed laparoscopically involves covering the hernial defect with prosthetic material. This differs from standard open hernia repair in that the prosthetic is placed on the undersurface of the floor of the inguinal canal (rather than on the anterior surface, as in open repair). The prosthetic material is fixed to the fascia with surgical staples.

Advantages

- Less postoperative pain
- Earlier return to work

Disadvantages

- Increased cost
- Lack of long-term follow-up studies

Laparoscopic Antireflux Surgery

Patients with symptomatic gastroesophageal reflux who fail medical therapy are candidates for antireflux surgery. Both the Nissen and Hill repairs can be performed laparoscopically with a high degree of success. (For details on the Nissen and Hill operations, see Chapter 31.)

Laparoscopic Colectomy

Laparoscopic colectomy has lagged behind the other laparoscopic procedures in widespread acceptance for the following reasons:

1. Questions persist on whether an adequate cancer operation can be done laparoscopically.
2. A learning curve exists, in which it takes 6 to 20 cases for surgeons to improve on operating time.
3. Worries persist about anecdotal reports of trocar site recurrences of cancer.

Some centers continue to offer laparoscopic colectomy for cancer. Others limit this procedure to patients operated on for benign disorders.

THORACOSCOPIC SURGERY

Chest surgery using thoracoscopy is rapidly developing. Pulmonary bleb resection with pleurodesis for recurrent pneumothorax is a procedure now done thoracoscopically. Lung biopsy can also be performed thoracoscopically.

CONTROVERSY: Major lung resections via the thoracoscope remain experimental. This is so because most thoracic surgeons respectfully fear pulmonary vascular injury that may not be controllable through the thoracoscope.

LIMITATIONS OF MINIMALLY INVASIVE SURGERY

The following are current limitations to performing minimally invasive surgery:

- Inadequate instrumentation
- Space limitations in major body cavities (limiting instrument maneuverability)
- Inability to deal with major blood vessels in rapid fashion

Eventually, improvements in technology will allow most procedures to be performed without large incisions.

2

PART

General Surgery

8
CHAPTER

Breast

BENIGN BREAST DISORDERS

As a glandular organ with hormonal receptors, the breast undergoes many changes throughout a woman's life. Parenchymal changes frequently appear as lumps or nodules. Benign breast lumps are commonly fibroadenomas (smooth and rubbery), cysts (round or ovoid), or fibrocystic masses. Benign breast lumps are much more common than cancers and are usually not precursors of breast cancer.

Because breast lumps cannot be entirely ensured as benign on physical exam, a tissue diagnosis is required. This may be obtained by means of fine-needle aspiration for cytology, a core biopsy (percutaneous), or an excisional biopsy. Exceptions not requiring a tissue diagnosis are multiple bilateral lumps and obvious fibroadenomas in women under 30 years of age.

CONTROVERSY: Long-term follow-up of presumed fibroadenomas (without a tissue diagnosis) in young women is controversial. Although cancer in this setting is rare, each missed cancer is associated with a high litigation rate.

Breast abscesses are frequently seen in lactating women. An early infection (redness and induration but no fluctuance) may respond to hot packs and oral antibiotics. A true abscess (fluctuant) needs to be incised and drained.

BREAST CANCER

Although benign breast disorders are very common, it is breast cancer that is feared by patients. One in 11 women will develop breast cancer.

The diagnosis and treatment of breast cancer have changed rapidly over the past decade. Physical examination (including self-exams) and mammography remain the mainstays of early diagnosis for breast cancer. Therefore, the workup of most breast disorders is triggered by either an examination (discovery of a breast lump) or an abnormal mammogram. In either situation, the office visit is commenced with a thorough history focusing on risk factors for the development of breast cancer.

Risk Factors

PEARL: Lobular carcinoma-in-situ (LCIS) is no longer considered a malignancy but is a marker for high risk for the development of invasive carcinoma. The following are risk factors for breast cancer:

- History of breast cancer in contralateral breast
- History of breast cancer in family
- Early menarche
- Late menopause
- Nulliparity

PEARL: The greatest risk factor for breast cancer is a history of breast cancer in the patient's contralateral breast.

Physical Examination

Physical examination of the breast begins with inspection, as follows:

- The patient is asked to raise her arms over her head, then to firmly push her hands onto the lateral aspect of the hips.
- During these maneuvers, the skin of the breast is observed for dimpling (a sign of underlying malignancy).

- The patient is then placed supine, and the breasts and axillae are palpated with the flat of the fingers.
- Any masses are noted for size, contour, mobility, and tenderness. Cancers tend to be firm or hard, irregular, and nontender. Fixation of a mass to the chest wall suggests a more advanced malignancy. Unilateral changes in a nipple or areola should raise suspicion of malignancy.
- Any nipple discharge is noted.

  - Bloody discharge is most frequently due to ductal papilloma and less frequently to carcinoma.
  - Green or brown fluid is often related to cystic lesions (benign).
  - Milky discharge (galactorrhea) is related to lactation, pharmaceutical agents (e.g., thorazine), or a prolactin-secreting pituitary tumor.

Mammography

Mammography is a complementary study to physical examination. Mammograms are used as a cancer screening tool in women over the age of 40 years.

In Women With Breast Lumps

Mammograms are obtained in women with breast lumps to study the surrounding parenchyma and the contralateral breast.

After bilateral mammograms, solitary breast lumps or dominant masses (in women with bilateral nodularity) are aspirated for cytology (fine-needle aspiration [FNA]). If the aspiration cytology is read as malignant, then breast cancer therapy can be planned. If it is read as benign it is generally followed by an excisional biopsy (removal of the lump) for a final pathologic diagnosis. **PEARL: The logic behind removal of breast lumps with benign cytology is to overcome the 5% to 10% false-negative cytologies due to "sampling error."**

CONTROVERSY: Some physicians are now willing to follow patients with benign needle or core biopsies.

In Women Without Breast Lumps

The workup of an abnormal mammogram in a woman with no palpable breast lump is more complicated. Certain characteristics on mammography are suggestive of malignancy:

- Asymmetric calcifications
- Stellate lesions
- Increased focal vascularity

If a mammographic lesion is suspicious, it can be evaluated with a **needle localization biopsy.** This is a procedure in which the radiologist inserts fine wires around the lesion and the surgeon removes the area as guided by the wires. The tissue obtained is then x-rayed to confirm removal of the suspicious image followed by pathologic examination.

Newer diagnostic modalities for breast lesions include ultrasound-guided biopsies and stereotactic-guided biopsies. These procedures are beginning to replace the needle localization technique for the biopsy of nonpalpable lesions.

Treatment

The treatment of breast cancer has evolved from inpatient care with radical surgery to multimodality outpatient care. The trend is to discover smaller and smaller tumors (nonpalpable <1 cm) detected by mammography. Small cancers are removed using radiographically guided techniques as described above. An axillary lymph node dissection or a sentinel node biopsy is performed for staging.

For palpable breast cancers smaller than 4 cm, there are two accepted therapies:

- Lumpectomy, axillary dissection, and breast irradiation
- Modified radical mastectomy

For palpable breast cancers larger than 4 cm, treatment is with modified radical mastectomy. With a modified radical mastectomy, the breast is removed down to the pectoralis fascia with preservation of the pectoralis muscles. The operation includes axillary node dissection (or sampling).

CONTROVERSY: In some cancer centers, lumpectomy (with histologic margins free of tumor) is now being used even with larger tumors.

Staging

Axillary node status helps stage the disease. Positive nodes are considered indicative of systemic malignancy and are an indication for the use of chemotherapy.

Complementary to the trend away from mastectomy is the trend toward **sentinel node biopsy.** The concept is that if the sentinel node (the first node in the local nodal drainage) is positive, then the patient is considered to have systemic disease and require chemotherapy, so the status of other nodes is irrelevant. Thus, a sentinel node biopsy could spare the patient the added trauma of full axillary node dissection. The sentinel node is identified by injection of a vital dye or radio-nuclear marker adjacent to the tumor.

Treatment Considerations

- Most breast cancers are invasive ductal carcinomas.
- Patients with medullary or lobular carcinomas have a better prognosis than those with invasive ductal carcinoma.
- Patients with positive axillary nodes are treated with axillary node dissection or radiation therapy to the axilla to control for local recurrence. These patients also receive chemotherapy.
- Patients with breast cancers that are positive for estrogen and progesterone receptors may also receive hormonal therapy, frequently with tamoxifen citrate (an estrogen receptor blocker).
- As the development of histologic and genetic markers for prognosis improves, patients with presumed poorer prognosis are being treated more aggressively. Treatment may include multi-drug chemotherapy, which wipes out the patient's bone marrow. Autologous bone marrow harvest and transplant has been developed for these patients.

Survival Rates

The following are the 5-year survival rates for the patient with breast cancer after accepted surgical or multimodality treatment:

Node-negative disease	90%
Node-positive disease	75%
Distant metastasis	30–40%

The great attention given to breast cancer has led to earlier detection and a concomitant improved outlook.

9
CHAPTER

Endocrine Disorders

This chapter deals primarily with conditions of the thyroid and parathyroid glands because they are common disorders. Although any good physician needs to be able to identify both hormone deficiency and hormone excess, the endocrine surgeon is usually dealing with either endocrine hyperfunction or endocrine malignancy.

The following are general principles regarding endocrinopathies:

- Be familiar with signs and symptoms of hormone excess (Table 9–1).
- Lab studies are important. (Biochemical confirmation is often by assay of hormone level.)

CENTRAL NECK ANATOMY

Thyroid means shield. The thyroid gland is shaped like a shield; the ancients probably thought that it was shielding the trachea. The anatomic landmarks of the central neck are presented briefly here:

- From anterior to posterior in the central neck are situated the thyroid, trachea, esophagus, and cervical vertebral column.
- There are two paired arteries—the superior thyroids (a branch of the external carotid) and the

Table 9–1. SIGNS AND SYMPTOMS
OF HORMONAL EXCESS

Tissue	Hormone	Signs and Symptoms
Pituitary	ACTH	Cushing's syndrome*
Pancreatic islet cells	Insulin	Hypoglycemia and blackouts
	Gastrin	Zollinger-Ellison syndrome†
	Glucagon	Mild diabetes, migrating necrolytic rash
Adrenal cortex	Cortisol	Cushing's syndrome*
	Aldosterone	Conn's syndrome
Adrenal medulla "pheochromocytoma"	Catecholamines	Severe hypertension
		Headaches
		Palpitations
Thyroid gland	Thyroid hormone	See Hyperthyroidism
Parathyroid gland	Parathyroid hormone	See Hyperparathyroidism

*Includes hypertension, truncal obesity, hirsutism, purple striations of abdominal skin, posterior cervical fat pad (buffalo hump), and sometimes diabetes mellitus.
†Severe peptic ulceration due to hypergastrinemia.

inferior thyroids (a branch of the thyrocervical trunk).
- The veins follow the arteries, except for the middle thyroid vein, which empties into the internal jugular vein on each side. (There is no middle thyroid artery.) **PEARL: The recurrent laryngeal nerves, the branches of the vagus that innervate the muscles of the larynx, run in the tracheoesophageal groove on each side of the neck. Injury to a recurrent nerve causes a permanent voice change, usually hoarseness.**
- The upper parathyroid glands are usually adjacent to the posterior surface of the upper pole of the thyroid.
- The lower parathyroid glands are often adjacent to the lower pole of the thyroid. Because they have

a common origin with the thymus, the lower parathyroids are frequently adjacent to or embedded in fat.

THYROID

The thyroid gland sets the metabolic stage for the entire body (Table 9–2). Hypothyroidism per se is never treated surgically. (Hyperthyroidism used to be treated surgically, but today it is usually treated by antithyroid medications followed by thyroid ablation with radioactive iodine.)

Thyroid Nodule

Thyroid nodules are common. **PEARL: You can differentiate a thyroid nodule from other central neck masses by the fact that a thyroid nodule moves up and down with swallowing.** Most nodules are benign.

Many imaging studies (ultrasound, MRI, CT scanning, and nuclear scanning) are available to provide information about the size and density of thyroid nodules. All algorithms for the evaluation of thyroid nodules lead to fine-needle aspiration (FNA) for cytology. Therefore, most authorities recommend reducing costs by avoiding imaging studies. Thus, thyroid nodules should by evaluated by FNA (Table 9–3).

**Table 9–2. SIGNS AND SYMPTOMS
OF THYROID IMBALANCE**

Hypothyroidism	Hyperthyroidism
Weight gain	Weight loss
Lethargy	Nervousness
Always feel cold	Always feel hot
Bradycardia	Tachycardia
Dry skin and hair	Exophthalmos
	Big appetite
	Tremors

Table 9–3. EVALUATION OF THYROID NODULES BY FNA

Result	Action
Inadequate specimen	Repeat FNA
Benign aspirate	Follow clinically with thyroid hormone–suppressive therapy
Suspicious for malignancy	Thyroid lobectomy with frozen section
Malignant	Thyroidectomy

Thyroid Cancer

Thyroid cancers are relatively common. Most affected patients have a good prognosis after surgical therapy (Table 9–4). The prognostic factors for thyroid cancer are:

- Cell type (papillary cancer = best prognosis; anaplastic = worst prognosis).
- Size of tumor (>5 cm = worse prognosis).
- Age (>45 = poorer prognosis).
- Sex (women have a slightly better prognosis than men).

Table 9–4. TYPES OF THYROID CANCER AND THEIR PROGNOSIS

Cell Type	Percent of Cases	Type of Metastasis	10-Year Survival After Surgery
Papillary	70	Local nodes	>90%
Follicular	15	Bone and lung	Dependent on invasiveness of tumor
Medullary	5	Central neck nodes	Dependent on nodal status
Anaplastic	5	Mostly local invasion	<5%

PEARL: Traditional chemotherapy and external-beam radiation are relatively useless against thyroid cancer.

PARATHYROID

There are four parathyroid glands—two upper and two lower. The lower parathyroid glands developed with the thymus from branchial arch 3 and descended past the upper parathyroids (from branchial arch 4) during development. Understanding this embryology helps the surgeon find the parathyroid glands. (Upper glands hug the posterior surface of the thyroid; lower glands are frequently adjacent to fat).

Primary Hyperparathyroidism

The parathyroid glands produce parathyroid hormone, which controls the serum calcium level. The old diagnostic mnemonic for primary hyperparathyroidism was "moans, bones, and stones:"

Moans = psychiatric complaints
Bones = bone pain
Stones = kidney stone

Now, however, most cases of primary hyperparathyroidism are picked up on mass electrolyte testing while the patient is asymptomatic. Moreover, many patients have more subtle symptoms such as joint pain, anxiety, muscle weakness, and memory loss.

PEARL: The most common cause of hypercalcemia is primary hyperparathyroidism. The most common cause of hypercalcemia in *hospitalized* patients is malignancy. Table 9–5 compares laboratory results from these two disorders.

Most patients (85%) with primary hyperparathyroidism have solitary adenomas. At operation, the surgeon finds one large gland (>8 mm) and three small or normal glands. Another 14% of affected patients have hyperplasia of all four glands, and 1% have double adenomas.

Table 9–5. PRIMARY HYPERPARATHYROIDISM VERSUS THE HYPERCALCEMIA OF MALIGNANCY

	Primary Hyperparathyroidism	Hypercalcemia of Malignancy
Ca^{2+}	↑	↑
PO_4	↓	Unreliable
Cl	↑	Unreliable
PTH	↑	Low or normal
PTHRP	↓	↑

PTH = parathyroid hormone; PTHRP = parathyroid hormone–related peptide.

Secondary and Tertiary Hyperparathyroidism

Secondary and tertiary hyperparathyroidism are seen in patients with chronic renal failure (CRF). CRF patients tend to have hyperphosphatemia and hypocalcemia, both of which increase the release of parathyroid hormone. Years of compensatory hyperparathyroid function can cause problems in the patient with CRF, including severe osteoporosis with bone pain and nephrocalcinosis with worsening of any residual renal function.

Patients with secondary hyperparathyroidism have very high parathyroid hormone levels but *normal serum calcium* (an equilibrium). CRF patients with tertiary hyperparathyroidism develop four autonomous parathyroid glands. Thus, the patient has a very high parathyroid hormone level and high calcium levels. Unlike those with primary hyperparathyroidism, patients with secondary and tertiary hyperparathyroidism tend to have four-gland hyperplasia.

THYROID AND PARATHYROID OPERATIONS

Operations on the thyroid and parathyroid glands are performed through low transverse cervical incisions (collar incisions), following these guidelines:

- The platysma muscle is divided, and superior and inferior subplatysmal flaps are developed.
- Two of the "strap muscles" (sternohyoid and sternothyroid) are retracted laterally, exposing the thyroid gland.
- For **thyroidectomy,** the vessels are individually divided between ligatures after identification of the ipsilateral recurrent laryngeal nerves.
- Care is taken to preserve the parathyroid glands. **PEARL: With parathyroid exploration, the pathology is determined by examining the size of each gland with the naked eye. Parathyroids larger than 8 mm in their greatest dimension are abnormal.**
- For **solitary adenoma,** remove the adenoma (enlarged gland), and take a 1-mm biopsy of another gland to prove that you saw normal parathyroids.
- For **four-gland hyperplasia,** the most common approach is to perform "3½-gland" parathyroidectomy, leaving a healthy 5- to 8-mm remnant of one gland on its vascular pedicle.
- An alternative procedure for four-gland hyperplasia is to perform a total (four-gland) parathyroidectomy and then mince half of one gland into 1-mm cubes and transplant them into the forearm (beneath the fascia).

Total parathyroidectomy plus transplantation was developed to avoid reoperation on the neck in patients in whom a remnant continued to grow, causing recurrent hyperparathyroidism. The disadvantage of this operation compared with 3½-gland resection is that you need a tissue bank (with frozen parathyroid gland from each patient) in case the first transplant fails to take.

MULTIPLE ENDOCRINE NEOPLASIA SYNDROMES

Multiple endocrine neoplasia (MEN) syndromes are rare familial constellations of endocrine tumors. Although these tumors are rare, they are common fodder for exam makers, so you need to know them (Table 9–6).

Table 9–6. CHARACTISTICS OF MULTIPLE ENDOCRINE NEOPLASIA SYNDROMES

MEN I	MEN IIA	MEN IIB or III*
Hyperpara-thyroidism	Medullary thyroid cancer	Medullary thyroid cancer
Pituitary adenomas	Pheochromo-cytoma	Pheochromo-cytoma
Pancreatic islet cell tumors	Hyperpara-thyroidism	Soft tissue tumors, a marfanoid habitus and sometimes megacolon

*Note that patients with MEN IIB (MEN III) do not have hyperparathyroidism.

PEARL: Note that in MEN I, all organs involved start with "p." But remember that it is the *organs,* because in MEN II there is pheochromocytoma, which starts with "p" but is not an organ.

MEN II babies can now be tested by molecular techniques for the gene for medullary thyroid cancer. Babies testing positive have a 100% chance of developing this cancer, so they undergo prophylactic thyroidectomy before the age of 10 years.

10
CHAPTER

Head and Neck Tumors

The head and neck are rich in lymphatic glands. Many neck masses are lymph nodes. The location of neck masses offers clues to their composition and origin. Central neck masses caudal to the thyroid cartilage are frequently thyroid nodules (see Chapter 9). Anterior triangle masses are most frequently lymph nodes. Occasionally, an adult presents with a branchial cleft cyst. **PEARL: The two major risk factors for oral, pharyngeal, and upper airway malignancies are tobacco and alcohol use.** A history of long-standing use of tobacco and alcohol in an adult with a neck mass raises the suspicion of malignancy.

WORKUP

The physical examination of patients with head and neck tumors is crucial and includes the following:

- Careful inspection and digital examination of the oral cavity
- A mirror exam of the pharynx and vocal cords
- Biopsies of areas of leukoplakia or erythroplasia of the oral cavity to rule out malignancy

Large anterior neck nodes are frequently due to metastatic cancer from oral, pharyngeal, nasopharyngeal, and upper airway malignancies. For the patient with a neck mass suspected to be metastatic cancer and when the physical exam does not reveal the primary tumor, continue the workup.

- Obtain and review posteroanterior and lateral chest x-rays.
- Obtain a fine-needle aspiration of the neck mass for cytologic evaluation; this frequently differentiates metastatic squamous-cell carcinoma from lymphoma or other pathology.
- If the fine-needle aspiration reveals metastatic squamous cell cancer, recommend a "triple endoscopy" to locate the primary tumor. **Triple endoscopy** includes flexible bronchoscopy, pharyngoscopy, and esophagoscopy. It is done not only to locate the primary tumor but also to rule out synchronous second primary tumors, which occur in 10 to 20% of these patients.

An adult with a neck mass who has poor dentition, or dental or oropharyngeal infection, may have "reactive" benign nodes in the neck. In such a patient with a recent history (<3 weeks) and small (<2 cm) soft nodes, a trial of antibiotic therapy is reasonable. If such a patient fails to respond to this therapy within 1 week, cancer must be sought. **PEARL: Large or firm to hard nodes are not compatible with infection but suggest malignancy.**

MANAGEMENT OF MALIGNANCIES

Oral and pharyngeal malignancies with definable anatomic margins are usually amenable to surgical resection.

Neck Dissection

Neck dissection is performed to remove presumed occult nodal metastases or obvious neck metastases in a resectable cancer case. A modified ipsilateral radical neck dissection may be indicated.

If the patient is clinically node-negative (i.e., no palpable nodes), the neck dissection includes en bloc removal of all lymphatics surrounding the internal jugular vein, with sparing of the internal jugular vein, the sternomastoid muscle, and the spinal accessory nerve.

If nodes are palpable (presumed nodal metastasis), the neck dissection includes en bloc removal of the internal jugular vein, sternomastoid muscle, and all lymphatics. This dissection spares only the spinal accessory nerve.

Radiation and Chemotherapy

Patients with specimen margins that are positive for cancer on pathologic exam generally receive postoperative radiation therapy. Multidrug chemotherapy plus radiation therapy is gaining acceptance as initial therapy for large head and neck cancers. Prospective comparisons between this approach and that of cancer surgery are in progress.

CONTROVERSY: Currently, either chemotherapy plus radiation or surgery is acceptable, and no strong data support one approach over the other.

Free-Flap Reconstruction

With radical cancer surgery of head and neck tumors, the surgical team must be adept at reconstructive procedures. A wide variety of reconstructive options are available, ranging from local rotational flaps to "free flaps" from other anatomic areas. Rotation flaps include latissimus dorsi and pectoralis major flaps. Free flaps include soft tissue such as the radial forearm flap and bone such as the fibular orthocutaneous flap for mandibular reconstruction. Free flaps depend on microvascular anastomoses for blood supply. Free-flap reconstruction therefore requires microvascular expertise. Reconstruction includes not only skin coverage but possibly mandibular and even pharyngeal reconstruction, depending on what has been resected.

It is not uncommon for these operations to result in impaired swallowing or an inadequate airway. Therefore, placement of a feeding tube or a tracheostomy is frequently required.

Several specific tumors are worthy of separate discussion.

LARYNGEAL TUMORS

PEARL: Long-standing hoarseness (>2 weeks) suggests neoplasm. Benign laryngeal neoplasms such as papillomas are frequently treated with laser vaporization.

The most common laryngeal malignancy is squamous cell carcinoma. Although radiation therapy alone is adequate treatment for small laryngeal tumors, the success rate drops in advanced lesions. Many laryngeal malignancies may be treated with radiation therapy, thus preserving voice, but laryngectomy for larger malignancies is sometimes necessary. This is a severely debilitating treatment. Partial laryngectomy has become more common, with resultant voice preservation.

Total laryngectomy leaves the patient with a permanent tracheostomy, which is accompanied by physiological as well as cosmetic concerns. Much research has been devoted to voice rehabilitation, with limited success.

SALIVARY GLAND TUMORS

PEARL: Enlargement of a salivary gland is neoplastic until proved otherwise. Most salivary gland tumors occur in the parotid gland. About 75% of parotid tumors are benign. In contrast, tumors of other salivary glands tend to be malignant.

Most parotid tumors occur in the superficial lobe, presenting as a mass beneath the ear lobe. Parotid tumors should be removed by means of a superficial lobectomy with careful dissection of the facial nerve. Facial nerve palsy in the face of a parotid tumor suggests squamous cell carcinoma. Table 10–1 lists the most common types of parotid tumors.

Table 10–1. COMMON TYPES OF PAROTID TUMORS*

Benign

Pleomorphic adenoma (formerly known as benign mixed
   tumor)
Warthin's tumor (papillary cystadenoma lymphomatosum)
Oxyphilic adenoma
Oncocytoma

Malignant

Mucoepidermoid carcinoma
Malignant mixed tumor
Acinic cell carcinoma
Adenocarcinoma
Adenoid cystic carcinoma
Squamous cell carcinoma (epidermoid carcinoma)

---

*Tumors are listed from most common to least common.

Invasive malignancies may require complete parotidectomy with sacrifice of the facial nerve. Great care
is taken to preserve the facial nerve during superficial
parotidectomy in contrast to what is necessary with benign tumors and smaller malignancies. The most commonly injured branch of the facial nerve with parotid
surgery is the marginal mandibular branch. Injury to
this branch results in unilateral lower lip droop.

11
CHAPTER

Acute Abdomen (Including Appendicitis)

Abdominal pain is a relatively common complaint of patients seen by general surgeons. Most cases are due to self-limiting conditions such as gastroenteritis. **PEARL: Two symptoms suggest disease of a surgical nature: abdominal pain that persists beyond 6 hours, and abdominal pain that is severe and began so suddenly that the patient noted the exact time.**

Abdominal pain comes in two forms—visceral and parietal.

- **Visceral pain** is evoked by distention or ischemia of an intra-abdominal organ (often a hollow viscus). The pain is referred to the midline and may be further localized according to the arterial blood supply (Table 11–1).
- **Parietal pain** localizes to the actual site of inflammation because of inflammation of the parietal peritoneum.

An **acute abdomen** occurs when a patient has abdominal pain and significant abdominal tenderness. The duration of the illness and concomitant signs of sepsis suggest a surgical condition. The patient's temperature and white blood cell (WBC) counts are used as guides, as are serial physical exams. Surgical causes of abdominal

Table 11–1. LOCALIZATION OF VISCERAL PAIN IN THE MIDLINE

Location	Blood Supply	Example
Epigastric	Celiac	Stomach and biliary tree
Periumbilical	Superior mesenteric artery	Small bowel and appendix
Suprapubic	Inferior mesenteric artery	Sigmoid colon and rectum

pain are often accompanied by oral temperatures higher than 100°F and WBC counts greater than 14,000.

COMMON CAUSES

The following are common causes of acute abdominal pain according to location.

Upper abdominal pain

- Acute cholecystitis
- Perforated ulcer
- Acute pancreatitis (nonsurgical disease)

Midabdominal pain

- Mesenteric ischemia
- Bowel obstruction

Lower abdominal pain

- Perforated sigmoid diverticulitis
- Acute appendicitis
- Pelvic inflammatory disease (in women) (nonsurgical disease)
- Ruptured ovarian cyst
- Ruptured ectopic pregnancy

If the patient has peritonitis (characterized by severe tenderness and guarding on physical exam), then exploratory laparotomy is indicated. "Free air" under the diaphragm on chest x-ray or upright abdominal films suggests perforation of a hollow viscus. **PEARL: Free air is most common with a perforated peptic ulcer and is less common with perforated appendicitis or perforated sigmoid diverticulitis.**

Individual diseases causing an acute abdomen (e.g., perforated ulcer, diverticulitis) are discussed in other appropriate chapters.

Acute Appendicitis

The best way to understand the difference between visceral and parietal pain is to consider acute appendicitis. This is a disease in which both types of pain occur. First, the appendix is obstructed (lymphoid tissue in babies, fecoliths in adults) and distends with mucus. This results in visceral pain (periumbilical). As the disease progresses, bacterial overgrowth in the lumen overcomes normal defenses and invades the appendiceal wall (acute appendicitis). Finally, the local infection results in inflammation of the adjacent parietal peritoneum, causing right lower quadrant pain (the well-known "pain shift" from periumbilical to right lower quadrant pain seen in appendicitis).

Signs and Symptoms

Acute appendicitis is most common in patients under the age of 20 years, but it can occur in any age group. Appendicitis most frequently results in fever (>100°F orally or 101° to 103°F rectally) and leukocytosis (WBCs 13,000 to 18,000). The temporal history is important. Pain occurs before any episodes of emesis. A history of emesis followed by lower abdominal pain makes appendicitis less likely. Patients with acute appendicitis are usually anorexic (i.e., a hungry patient is unlikely to have acute appendicitis). Profuse diarrhea is unusual in acute appendicitis.

Treatment

Acute appendicitis is treated with appendectomy. This is most frequently performed with a small transverse incision in the right lower quadrant. Traditionally, the surgeon identifies **McBurney's point** to guide incision placement. McBurney's point is located two thirds of the distance along a line drawn from the umbilicus to the right anterior superior iliac spine.

Laparoscopic appendectomy has recently become popular. Whether open or laparoscopic surgery is done, most patients are discharged by the third postoperative day after appendectomy for acute (but not perforated) appendicitis.

Mesenteric Ischemia

PEARL: Severe abdominal pain out of proportion to physical findings suggests mesenteric ischemia. This condition is an emergency requiring operation or a mesenteric angiogram followed by appropriate therapy. If the patient presents within 4 hours of the onset of pain, one should proceed with a mesenteric angiogram.

If the mesenteric angiogram suggests nonocclusive, low-flow ischemia, then the treatment is nonsurgical. This condition is usually due to a low cardiac output. The patient should be moved to an intensive care unit, and a pulmonary artery catheter should be inserted. Fluid and pharmacological therapy (e.g. dobutamine) should be instituted to increase cardiac output and thus improve blood flow to the intestines. Table 11–2 lists treatments for mesenteric ischemia based on etiology.

Table 11–2. THERAPY FOR MESENTERIC ISCHEMIA

Cause	Treatment
Low flow	Mesenteric papaverine infusion
	Cardiac support (dobutamine)
Superior mesenteric artery embolus	Embolectomy
Superior mesenteric artery thrombus	Thrombectomy or thrombolytic therapy
Venous thrombosis	Venous thrombectomy Anticoagulation

In patients with mesenteric ischemia, nonviable bowel is resected. To avoid short bowel syndrome, questionable small bowel is sometimes left in-situ to be reexamined at 24 hours with a "second look" procedure.

PREPARATIONS FOR SURGERY

Patients requiring surgery for an acute abdomen should be rapidly prepared for surgery. To decrease morbidity, the following measures should be taken:

- Rapid fluid resuscitation (more than 1 liter per hour IV crystalloid solution, if necessary)
- Placement of Foley catheter to ensure perfusion of vital organs (urine output depends on renal perfusion)
- Type and screen or type and crossmatch for blood, depending on patient's condition, hemoglobin level, and magnitude of anticipated surgery
- Administration of appropriate IV antibiotics
- The surgeon should discuss all possible diagnoses and treatments with the patient and family before surgery. This is particularly true if a colostomy is a possible procedure. In addition, many patients with peritonitis have a long recovery period. Intraoperative placement of a feeding tube should be considered if long-term nutritional support is a possibility.

12
CHAPTER

Stomach and Duodenum

The stomach is the site of a myriad of disorders, both benign and malignant. The duodenum is the site of duodenal ulcer and is rarely the site of a malignancy. The most common symptoms that point toward gastroduodenal disease are:

- Epigastric pain (dyspepsia)
- Upper gastrointestinal (GI) bleeding

The gastric mucosa lives in a delicate balance between damage by its own hydrochloric acid and protection by its intrinsic defenses (e.g., mucus, rapid cell turnover, prostaglandins). Factors that tip the balance toward injury and disease include aspirin, nonsteroidal anti-inflammatory drugs (NSAIDs), alcohol, critical illness (stress), and *Helicobacter pylori* infection.

H. pylori infection of the gastric antrum is the most common infection in the Western world. **Gastritis** is inflammation of the gastric mucosa. *H. pylori* infection always results in gastritis. Other causes of gastritis include NSAIDs and alcohol. Gastritis is treated medically and almost never requires surgical therapy.

PEPTIC ULCER

Background

For many decades our entire understanding of the pathophysiology of peptic ulcer focused on gastric acid hypersecretion. When populations of ulcer patients were studied, however, many patients did *not* secrete abnormally high levels of acid. Despite this, medical therapy, such as antacids, H_2-blockers and H^+-K^+ pump inhibitors, was developed to combat acid injury to the mucosa.

Similarly, the history of anti-ulcer surgery revolves around acid secretion. We still accept acid injury as a major part of the ulcer puzzle. However, in 1982, the discovery of the "ulcer bacterium" *H. pylori* changed our understanding of the disease and has had a profound impact on the medical therapy for the disease.

Pathogenesis

Peptic ulcers are inflammatory lesions of the stomach or duodenum associated with local loss of mucosa. The most common ulcerogenic agent is *H. pylori*. The pathophysiology of *H. pylori*-associated peptic ulcer is unclear. Possible mechanisms include *H. pylori* effects on gastrin or acid production and effects on immune cells.

NSAIDs are the second most common ulcerogenic agents. NSAIDs (including aspirin) cause a twofold injurious effect:

- Diminished production of protective prostaglandins
- Direct cell membrane injury to gastric and duodenal mucosal cells.

Duodenal

Most duodenal ulcers occur in the first portion of the duodenum. Ulcers on the posterior wall can erode the gastroduodenal artery and cause massive upper GI bleeding. They occasionally erode into the pancreas and are thus an unusual cause of acute pancreatitis.

Anterior and lateral duodenal ulcers are at risk for perforation into the peritoneal cavity. This causes excruciating abdominal pain owing to the acid burn of the peritoneum. **PEARL: Perforated gastric or duodenal ulcers are surgical emergencies.**

Gastric

Gastric ulcers frequently occur on the lesser curvature but may occur anywhere in the stomach. In contrast to duodenal ulcers, gastric ulcers may be malignant (Table 12–1). **PEARL: Because of the chance of malignancy, the rim of all gastric ulcers should be biopsied when they are identified endoscopically.**

Treatment

Peptic ulcer is primarily a medical disease. Medical therapy may include antacids, H_2 blockers, H^+-K^+ pump blockers (omeprazol), and antibiotics to eradicate *H. pylori*. The following are indications for surgery for peptic ulcer:

- GI bleeding (requiring more than 2 units of blood)
- Perforation
- Pyloric obstruction (due to edema and inflammation)
- Failure of medical management

Many operations have been devised to combat ulcer. They work by decreasing acid output.

Table 12–1. COMPARISON OF GASTRIC AND DUODENAL ULCERS

	H. pylori-Positive	Healed at 6 weeks on Medical Therapy	Risk of Cancer
Gastric	60–80%	80%	+
Duodenal	>90%	>90%	−

- Vagotomy decreases acid output by 40%.
- Antrectomy removes gastrin-producing cells, again inhibiting acid output.

Lester Dragstedt, surgeon and physiologist, popularized vagotomy for peptic ulcer in the mid-twentieth century. When he discovered that vagotomy alone impaired gastric emptying, he added an emptying procedure. The two types of emptying procedures are pyloroplasty (which renders the pyloric sphincter incompetent) and gastrojejunostomy (anastomosis between the stomach and proximal jejunum). Thus, vagotomy plus an emptying procedure is an acceptable operation for peptic ulcer. The combination of vagotomy and antrectomy, however, has been the surgical gold standard operation for peptic ulcer for decades.

During the 1970s and 1980s, a new operation was developed for peptic ulcer. This is known as **highly selective vagotomy** or **parietal cell vagotomy.** In this procedure, the vagal branches to the stomach are cut along the lesser curvature. The branches to the antrum are left intact. Thus, acid-producing (proximal) stomach is denervated while the motor unit (antrum) remains functional.

With antrectomy or subtotal gastrectomy, the proximal GI tract must be reconstructed. The means of GI reconstruction are the same for resection for gastric ulcer as for cancer (see Gastric Cancer).

The various anti-ulcer operations differ in outcome. The surgeon has to consider the complication rate with the rate of recurrent ulcer (Table 12–2). Finally, to state the obvious, when operating for acute bleeding ulcer, the bleeding blood vessel is oversewn (sutured) in the ulcer itself. When operating for perforated ulcer, the perforation is closed with sutures. If the perforation is patched or plugged with omentum, it is called a Graham patch.

GASTRIC CANCER

The incidence of adenocarcinoma of the stomach has declined over this century. Because the stomach is a sizable, distensible bag, these tumors tend to be large before becoming symptomatic. Large tumors cause early satiety. Gastric cancers may also cause low-grade GI bleeding (commonly found as fecal occult blood).

Table 12–2. COMPLICATIONS OF
ANTI-ULCER SURGERY

Operation	Physiological Complications*	Ulcer Recurrence
Vagotomy and pyloroplasty	+	5–10%
Vagotomy and antrectomy	+ +	3–5%
Subtotal gastrectomy	+ + +	3–5%
Parietal cell vagotomy†	−	5–20%

*Includes diarrhea and vasomotor symptoms such as diaphoresis and palpitations. This is sometimes called **dumping syndrome.**
†Involves leaving the vagus trunks intact but cutting vagal branches to the body of the stomach (hence removing vagal stimulation of parietal cells).

Gastric cancer comes in two forms: fungating and infiltrating. The infiltrating type grows laterally within the gastric wall. This type is more lethal and is sometimes called linitis plastica or leather-bottle stomach.

Treatment and Prognosis

Treatment for gastric cancer is surgical resection. Large cancers, mid-body tumors, and proximal tumors usually require a total gastrectomy.

CONTROVERSY: Asian literature suggests that radical gastrectomy, including splenectomy and meticulous celiac node dissection, improves the prognosis of gastric cancer patients. American literature does not support this.

Reconstructions of GI continuity after partial gastrectomy are named for the German surgical pioneer, Theodor Billroth. A Billroth I is an anastomosis between the proximal gastric remnant and the duodenum (Fig. 12–1). A Billroth II involves closing the duodenal stump and anastomosing the gastric remnant to the proximal jejunum (Fig. 12–2). Finally, after total gastrectomy, most reconstructions are from esophagus to jejunum (Roux-en-Y) (Fig. 12–3), named after the Swiss surgeon, César Roux.

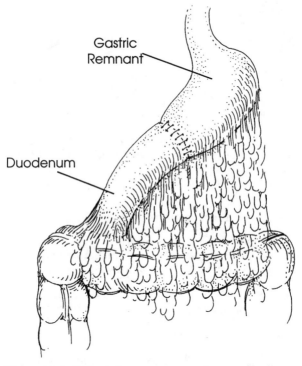

Figure 12–1. Billroth I reconstruction after partial gastrectomy.

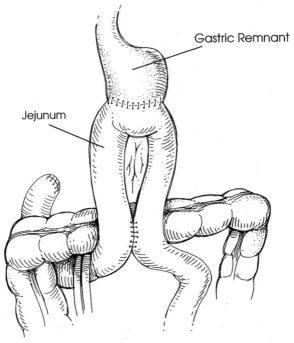

Figure 12–2. Billroth II gastrojejunostomy after partial gastrectomy. Note that the duodenal stump is oversewn.

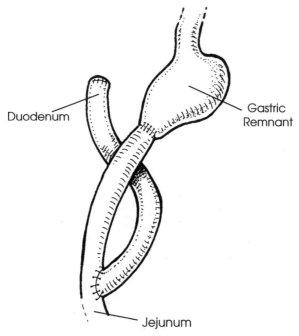

Figure 12–3. Roux-en-Y reconstruction after subtotal gastrectomy.

Small antral cancers may be treated with subtotal gastrectomy. Subtotal gastrectomy leaves a small residual proximal gastric pouch.

PEARL: The two most important prognostic factors in gastric cancer are depth of gastric wall invasion and lymph node status.

- The 5-year survival rate after surgery for gastric cancer is less than 10%.
- In stage I (node-negative and no transmural invasion) gastric cancer, the 5-year survival rate is 15 to 30%.

13
CHAPTER

Liver, Spleen, and Biliary Tree

THE LIVER

The liver is the largest solid organ in the abdomen. An imaginary plane through the gallbladder bed to the inferior vena cava divides the liver into left and right lobes. The falciform ligament divides the left lobe into a left lateral and left medial segment. The left hepatic duct and the right hepatic duct join to form the common hepatic duct (Fig. 13–1). The cystic duct from the gallbladder drains into the common hepatic duct, becoming the common bile duct. Calot's triangle is formed by the liver edge, the common hepatic duct, and the cystic duct. The triangle contains the cystic artery.

The hepatic artery (a branch of the celiac artery) carries oxygenated blood to the liver. It supplies 25% of hepatic blood. The portal vein brings nutrient-enriched venous blood from the intestines to the liver. The portal vein supplies 75% of hepatic blood flow.

Although the hepatic artery brings valuable oxygen to hepatocytes, it is portal venous blood that brings the materials needed by the liver to perform its incredible role as a factory. Protein synthesis in the liver provides albumin and a variety of blood clotting factors.

Glycogen is produced and stored by the liver. Phos-

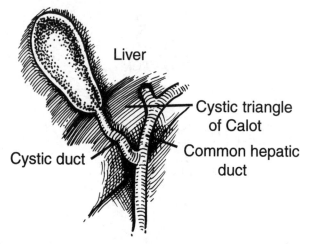

Figure 13–1. Biliary ductal anatomy including Calot's triangle (see text).

pholipids and cholesterol are produced in the liver. Cholesterol is the basic building block for corticosteroid hormone production by various endocrine organs. Bilirubin is the end product of hemoglobin breakdown. Unconjugated bilirubin is transported in plasma. The liver concentrates and "conjugates" bilirubin (mostly as glucuronides), which is needed for digestion and absorption of fats. Venous blood returns from the liver to the inferior vena cava via hepatic veins located on the posterior surface of the liver.

In addition to synthetic and secretory functions, the liver is a major part of the reticuloendothelial system. Kupffer's cells are phagocytic and contribute to the filtration and detoxification functions of the liver.

Liver Failure

Understanding normal hepatic function facilitates a better understanding of hepatic failure. **PEARL: The most common cause of liver failure in the Western world is chronic alcohol damage with resultant cirrhosis.** Other causes of liver failure are hepatitis, repeated episodes of shock (ischemia), acetaminophen toxicity, replacement of hepatic substance by tumor, and acute ethanol damage (alcoholic hepatitis).

Table 13–1 lists the manifestations of liver failure based on normal hepatic function. In addition to these manifestations, some events cascade into more signs and symptoms, such as ecchymoses from the coagulopathy, ascites in part from hypoalbuminemia, and severe pruritus due to hyperbilirubinemia.

In patients with cirrhosis, hepatic parenchyma is replaced by scar tissue. This results in an increased resistance to portal blood flow (portal hypertension). Portal hypertension can lead to the formation of esophageal varices. These dilated submucosal veins in the distal esophagus are prone to rupture, resulting in life-threatening hematemesis (discussed in further detail in Chap 31).

> **CONTROVERSY: Many lab tests called liver function tests really don't measure liver function. For example, the serum transaminase levels are really a measure of cytotoxicity or damage to hepatocytes. The prothrombin time and the serum albumin levels better reflect liver function.**

Table 13–1. MANIFESTATIONS OF LIVER FAILURE COMPARED WITH NORMAL LIVER FUNCTION

Normal Function	Liver Failure Manifestation
Uptake and secretion of bile	Jaundice
Production of clotting factors	Coagulopathy
Synthesis of albumin	Hypoalbuminemia (contributes to ascites formation)
Detoxification of portal blood	Encephalopathy

Hepatic Tumors

Most hepatic tumors are metastatic deposits—most often from GI tract malignancies. Primary hepatic malignancies include hepatoma and cholangiocarcinoma (rare). In Asia, hepatoma (liver cancer) is associated with hepatic parasites. In the United States, hepatoma is associated with cirrhosis. Hepatoma and cholangiocarcinoma are both associated with a very poor prognosis.

Solitary liver metastases from a colon cancer may be resected, resulting in a 5-year survival rate of 25%. These are major operations, often associated with significant blood loss. When metastases are on the liver surface, they can be "wedge"-resected. Deeper lesions require formal liver lobectomy. Bilobar metastases are a contraindication to surgery.

Clinical research is currently being conducted to evaluate the efficacy of cryotherapy (freezing) of liver tumors.

THE SPLEEN

The spleen is an organ of the immune system. It sits high in the left upper quadrant, posterolateral beneath the left hemidiaphragm. The splenic artery is a branch of the celiac axis. Also, short gastric arteries are between the spleen and the fundus of the stomach. The splenic vein and the superior mesenteric vein join to form the portal vein.

The spleen acts as a filter for circulating blood. Aged blood cells of all types and platelets are sequestered and destroyed in the spleen. It is thus easy to see why hyperfunction (hypersplenism) can result in anemia or thrombocytopenia.

Hemolytic anemias may be congenital or acquired. In congenital hemolytic anemias, distorted or structurally abnormal red blood cells are destroyed. Splenectomy allows acceptable red cell counts, but it obviously does nothing for the intrinsic red cell abnormality.

Surgery

Indications

- Spherocytosis
- Elliptocytosis
- Hemolytic anemia (after failure of corticosteroid therapy)
- Idiopathic thrombocytopenic purpura (after failure of corticosteroid therapy)

Idiopathic thrombocytopenic purpura (ITP) is an autoimmune disorder manifested by platelet destruction. When platelet counts get very low (< 20,000), spontaneous hemorrhage may occur. Initial therapy is with corticosteroids. Patients not responding to corticosteroids usually recover after splenectomy.
PEARL: The most common indication for splenectomy is traumatic splenic rupture. Patients with splenic injuries are treated based on the magnitude of the injury. Subcapsular bleeds (on CT scan) may be observed. Small capsular tears may be repaired. Deep parenchymal laceration or rupture is treated with splenectomy.

Pediatric surgeons have practiced nonoperative and operative **splenic salvage** (efforts to repair and save an injured spleen) for decades. Recently, surgeons have been observing adults with low-grade injuries.

Complications

The complications of splenectomy are similar whether performed open or laparoscopically. These include pancreatitis (from operative injury to the tail of the pancreas), thrombocytosis, and postsplenectomy sepsis. Postsplenectomy sepsis is characterized by an increased susceptibility to infection particularly from encapsulated organisms. This syndrome led to the concept of splenic salvage in children.

THE BILIARY TREE

For the surgeon, the liver and biliary tree are most commonly dealt with for biliary stones or malignancy.

It is important to keep your terminology straight when discussing the biliary tree (Table 13–2).

Biliary Stones

Within bile, there is a delicate balance between cholesterol, lecithin, and bile salt concentrations. If bile becomes supersaturated with cholesterol, crystals may form, leading to stone formation. Hemolytic conditions may lead to the formation of black "pigment" stones. Biliary stasis in an atonic gallbladder is also believed to contribute to stone formation.

Gallstones cause trouble for millions of people, as illustrated in Table 13–3. Note that conditions due to gallstones are generally treated surgically. **PEARL: Asymptomatic gallstones do not require cholecystectomy.** Medical therapy of gallstones, "dissolution," has been a dismal failure.

Acute Cholecystitis

The pathophysiology of acute cholecystitis is obstruction of a hollow viscus, similar to that of acute appendicitis. With a stone in the cystic duct, the gallbladder cannot empty. Mucus production by the gallbladder epithelium leads to further distention. Small numbers of bacteria that are frequently present in gallbladders containing stones begin to multiply. Eventually, bacterial

Table 13–2. BILIARY TREE TERMINOLOGY

Term	Definition
Cholecyst (prefix)	Gallbladder
Cholecystitis	Inflammation or infection of gallbladder
Cholangio (prefix)	Bile duct
Cholangiogram	X-ray of bile duct
Cholangitis	Inflammation or infection within bile duct
Cholelithiasis	Stones in biliary tree

Table 13–3. CLINICAL CONDITIONS CAUSED BY GALLSTONES ACCORDING TO POSITION

Position of Gallstone	Clinical Problem
Periodic impaction in cystic duct	Biliary colic (right upper quadrant pain)
Permanent impaction in cystic duct	Hydrops of the gallbladder or, more commonly, acute cholecystitis (due to bacteria)
Impaction in common bile duct	Jaundice or cholangitis (if bacteria are present)
Impaction at ampulla of Vater	Jaundice, cholangitis, or pancreatitis

numbers are so great that the edematous gallbladder wall becomes infected. Acute cholecystitis is the result.

Patients with acute cholecystitis usually have right upper quadrant or epigastric pain, fever, and leukocytosis. **PEARL: In acute cholecystitis, you may elicit Murphy's sign. With the examining hand pressing the right upper quadrant, the patient is asked to take a deep breath. The descending diaphragm pushes the liver and gallbladder to the examiner's hand, eliciting pain (which on exam is known as tenderness).**

Acute cholecystitis is a surgical condition, most often treated by cholecystectomy.

CONTROVERSY: Some surgeons first treat the patient with IV antibiotics and fasting to minimize inflammation. This may allow laparoscopic cholecystectomy.

The standard therapy for acute cholecystitis remains IV hydration followed by cholecystectomy, usually within hours of admission to the hospital.

Acute Cholangitis

Acute cholangitis is an emergency. **PEARL: Charcot's triad is jaundice, fever, and right upper quadrant pain,** which is considered pathognomonic for cholangitis. Untreated, septic shock may ensue, causing hypotension and confusion. With Charcot's triad, this syndrome is known as Reynolds' pentad.

The treatment algorithm for cholangitis has changed in the past 10 years. Now, rather than emergency surgery with common bile duct exploration, the treatment is coordinated between gastroenterologist and surgeon. IV hydration and IV antibiotics remain mainstays of therapy. To decompress the obstructed, infected duct, an endoscopic retrograde cholangiopancreatogram with papillotomy (ERCP) is performed. With the scope in place in the duodenum, a papillotomy is performed using a wire passed through the instrument port of the endoscope. The impacted stone or stones can usually be extracted or may pass spontaneously, thus alleviating the infection. Later, an elective laparoscopic cholecystectomy may be performed to prevent future complications of gallstones. Here, modern technology has converted a huge open operation into two lesser invasive procedures.

BILIARY IMAGING

The liver and biliary tree may be imaged by means of a variety of techniques. Ultrasound is noninvasive and relatively inexpensive. It has a sensitivity of over 90% for gallstones and can also assess hepatic size, hepatic masses, and biliary tract dilatation. CT is more expensive and less sensitive for gallstones. However, CT provides a broad view of intra-abdominal structures and, unlike ultrasound, is not impeded by bowel gas. ERCP (described previously) and percutaneous cholangiography offer superb ductal images and can help assess stone versus tumor in cases of obstruction.

The HIDA (dimethyl iminodiacetic acid) scan (a radionuclide study) is the gold standard for ruling out acute cholecystitis. In this study, the patient is given an IV radionuclide, which is then taken up by the liver and secreted into the biliary tree. If the cystic duct is blocked by a stone, there will be no gallbladder image and the radionuclide will empty from the biliary tree to the duodenum. This would constitute a **positive study,** that is, no gallbladder image, for acute cholecystitis.

14
CHAPTER

Pancreas

The pancreas is both an **exocrine** (secreting into ducts) and **endocrine** (secreting into the vasculature) organ.

The exocrine function of the pancreas is to produce and secrete digestive enzymes, which are emptied through the pancreatic duct into the duodenum. Exocrine failure of the pancreas results in malabsorption of fats and steatorrhea.

The pancreatic islet cells contain the endocrine cells. These cells produce specific hormones including insulin, gastrin, and somatostatin. Endocrine failure is best known by the development of diabetes mellitus.

As with other organs, the surgeon is often called on to treat either inflammation or tumor. Inflammation of the pancreas is known as pancreatitis.

ACUTE PANCREATITIS

Signs and Symptoms

The patient with acute pancreatitis presents with the following symptoms:

- Epigastric pain often accompanied by nausea and vomiting. The pain is frequently severe and sometimes radiates to the back.
- Pain often out of proportion to physical findings (although most patients have some epigastric tenderness). Note: do not confuse pain, which is a

symptom, with tenderness, a sign elicited by physical examination.

- Elevations of the serum amylase and the serum lipase (usually).
- Low-grade fever and leukocytosis (WBCs [white blood cells] 12,000 to 15,000).

Hemorrhagic pancreatitis (a severe form of the disease) characterized by retroperitoneal hemorrhage is rare in the United States. When it occurs the patient may have flank ecchymosis (Grey Turner sign) or umbilical ecchymosis (Cullen's sign).

Causes

PEARL: The two most common causes of pancreatitis are alcohol abuse and gallstones. Why some people are prone to alcoholic pancreatitis and others are not is unknown. Alcoholic pancreatitis may be due to direct acinar cell injury resulting from alcohol plus indirect effects. Indirect contributions to inflammation may be due to increased pancreatic secretions and sphincter of Oddi spasm due to alcohol.

The mechanism of gallstone pancreatitis is better understood. Gallstones temporarily trapped at the ampulla of Vater can cause pancreatic ductal obstruction and resultant ductal hypertension. This obstruction may then result in pancreatic enzyme leakage into the pancreatic parenchyma with resultant cell injury and inflammation.

Treatment

The mainstays of treatment for acute pancreatitis are IV hydration and bowel rest. Although use of a nasogastric tube is traditional, its use has never been shown to be of benefit with this disease. Many physicians use a nasogastric tube selectively for patients who are vomiting.

PEARL: H_2-blockers and antibiotics have not been shown to affect the course of acute pancreatitis.

Prognosis

It is possible to predict to some degree the patient's prognosis based on Ranson's criteria (Table 14–1).

Most patients have mild pancreatitis, which is short lived and self-limiting. A patient with more severe disease may develop a complication of the disease. Surgery for acute pancreatitis is reserved for patients with a complication of the disease. The two most common complications of the disease are pseudocyst formation and the development of pancreatic abscess.

PSEUDOCYST

A **pseudocyst** is a fluid collection. It is not a true cyst because its walls have no epithelial lining. The walls of a pseudocyst are the outer surfaces of surrounding organs (e.g., stomach, bowel). Patients with pancreatic pseudocysts may have pain or may be pain-free, and

Table 14–1. RANSON'S CRITERIA FOR ACUTE PANCREATITIS*

On admission
Age >55 years
Glucose >200
WBCs >16,000
Lactic dehydrogenase elevation
Aspartate transaminase (AST) >2 times normal

At 48 hours
HCT $\downarrow$>10%
Calcium <8.0
Po_2 <60
Metabolic acidosis
Blood urea nitrogen (BUN) increasing

*Three or more factors present equals a 60% mortality rate; six or more factors equals an 80% mortality rate.

they may have a palpable epigastric mass. The serum amylase frequently remains elevated.

The pseudocyst is frequently discovered by ultrasound or CT scan. Rupture is a feared complication; for this reason pseudocysts are drained electively. This is usually done surgically with an anastomosis of the pseudocyst to an adjacent hollow viscus (stomach or small bowel).

CONTROVERSY: Recently percutaneous drainage of pancreatic pseudocysts has gained some favor.

PANCREATIC ABSCESS

Patients with pancreatic abscess have signs of systemic illness with prolonged fever and leukocytosis. The abscess may involve retroperitoneal fat manifested as fat necrosis, phlegmon formation, or both. It may also involve necrotic pancreas.

Abscesses are best defined by CT scan.

Treatment is surgical debridement and drainage. Patients may require repeated debridements, and pancreatic abscess can ultimately be a lethal disease.

CHRONIC PANCREATITIS

Patients with chronic pancreatitis commonly present with unremitting epigastric pain (sometimes radiating to the back). The pancreatitis may result in exocrine (malabsorption) or endocrine (diabetes) failure. Because of chronic pain, affected patients are frequently dependent on narcotics.

Chronic pancreatitis involves scarring of pancreatic parenchyma and pancreatic ductal dilatation. The duct and ductules may be calcified, possibly appearing on plain x-rays as diffuse calcific stippling in the pancreatic region. An endoscopic retrograde cholangiopancreatogram (ERCP) is done to evaluate the pancreatic duct. A diffusely dilated duct or a duct with segmental dilatation (chain of lakes phenomenon) may be seen.

Surgical drainage of the calcified, dilated pancreatic duct (longitudinal pancreaticojejunostomy) results in pain relief in about 75% of cases. The duration of pain relief from surgical drainage of the pancreatic duct is variable.

CONTROVERSY: The reliability of pain relief from surgical therapy for chronic pancreatitis is in question.

PANCREATIC TUMORS

Patients with pancreatic cancer most frequently present with epigastric or upper mid-back pain or both. Pancreatic pain is sometimes relieved when the patient sits forward.

If the tumor is in the head of the pancreas, the bile duct may be obstructed, resulting in jaundice. If the pancreatic mass is large, it may impinge on the duodenum, resulting in nausea and vomiting. Weight loss generally indicates advanced, incurable disease.

Treatment

Fewer than 20% of patients have tumors confined to the pancreas at the time of diagnosis, which are thus resectable for cure. Because the pancreas and duodenum share an arterial blood supply, one cannot be removed without the risk of ischemia to the other. That is why carcinoma of the head or body of the pancreas is treated by pancreaticoduodenectomy (also known as Whipple's operation).

In Whipple's operation, most of the pancreas is resected (leaving the tail), and the duodenum is removed enbloc. This leaves an open common bile duct end, an open distal stomach, an open pancreatic duct (in the tail), and an open proximal jejunum. The integrity of the GI tract is restored with three anastomoses: stomach to jejunum, bile duct to jejunum, and pancreatic duct to stomach or jejunum. (Fig. 14–1).

Postoperatively, with most of the pancreas and the duodenum out, patients are given oral pancreatic enzymes to aid in digestion. Few patients are rendered diabetic after the Whipple procedure. This major

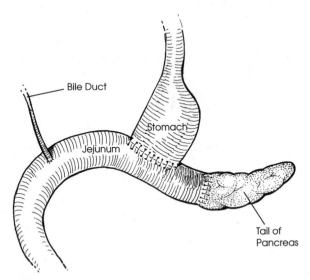

Figure 14–1. This illustration shows one acceptable surgical reconstruction after a pancreaticoduodenectomy (Whipple).

operation is accompanied by a complication rate of 40 to 60%. A serious complication is leakage of the pancreatic anastomosis. Whipple's operation has an operative mortality rate of 3 to 10%. The 5-year survival rate after this procedure for carcinoma of the pancreas is a dismal 5%.

Palliative Surgery

Patients with advanced disease may benefit from palliative surgery. An obstructed bile duct may be decompressed with a bypass procedure such as choledochojejunostomy. Similarly, an obstructed duodenum may be bypassed with a gastrojejunostomy. Palliative surgery for pancreatic cancer is associated with about a 4- to 18-month survival period, depending partly on the extent of the cancer.

**Table 14–2. SYNDROMES RESULTING
FROM ISLET CELL TUMORS**

Tumor	Hormone	Syndrome
Gastrinoma	Gastrin	Zollinger-Ellison (severe peptic ulcers)
Insulinoma	Insulin	Spells due to intermittent hypoglycemia

Islet Cell Tumors

Islet cell tumors are uncommon. They result in hypersecretion of hormones with resultant syndromes (Table 14–2). Islet cell tumors are **enucleated** from the pancreas; thus major pancreatic resections are not usually required.

15
CHAPTER

Small Bowel

SMALL-BOWEL OBSTRUCTION

The most common surgical disorder of the small bowel is **small-bowel obstruction.** All other surgical disorders of the small bowel are uncommon.

Signs and Symptoms

- Mid-abdominal pain coming in "waves" as peristalsis pushes against the obstructed point
- Nausea and vomiting
- Distended and tympanitic abdomen
- Dehydration
- Dilated small bowel with air-fluid levels seen on plain films of the abdomen

With obstructed bowel, net fluid movement may be from the bowel wall to the lumen (secretory) rather than the usual reverse (absorptive) path. This combination of fluid loss via vomiting and "third spacing" (an increase in interstitial fluid due to inflammation) results in dehydration. Thus, patients require fluid resuscitation and electrolyte repletion before surgery.

Treatment

Partial small-bowel obstruction is present if gas is in the colon and the patient still passes flatus. This obstruction can be treated with a nasogastric tube, bowel rest, and IV hydration.

Complete small-bowel obstruction is a dangerous situation and must be treated surgically. In a patient with prior abdominal surgery, the most common cause of small-bowel obstruction is adhesions, followed by incarcerated hernia. All other causes are a distant third. Table 15–1 compares the causes of small-bowel obstruction with colon obstruction.

Strangulation

Small bowel that is incarcerated in a hernia or twisted internally (e.g., volvulus around an adhesion) may jeopardize its blood supply. This is known as "strangulation" of the bowel. Strangulated bowel quickly becomes gangrenous and results in peritonitis, a potentially fatal condition. This is why small-bowel obstruction is treated urgently with operation (most commonly with lysis of adhesions).

OTHER SMALL-BOWEL DISORDERS

Tumors

Small-bowel tumors include:

- Lipomas
- Leiomyomas
- Polyps
- Adenocarcinoma (rare)

Table 15–1. CAUSES OF SMALL-BOWEL OBSTRUCTION (SBO) COMPARED WITH CAUSES OF COLON OBSTRUCTION

SBO	Frequency	Colon Obstruction
Adhesions	Most common	Colon cancer
Hernia	Less common	Sigmoid diverticulitis
All others	Least common	Sigmoid volvulus

Patients with small-bowel tumors often present with melena or intermittent rectal bleeding. These tumors rarely cause obstruction. They usually are not suspected until the patient has had negative upper and lower endoscopy as a workup for gastrointestinal (GI) bleeding.

Meckel's Diverticulum

Meckel's diverticulum is a congenital true diverticulum of the distal ileum. It is a remnant of the omphalomesenteric duct and most frequently occurs in the most distal two feet of ileum.

Most patients with Meckel's diverticulum are asymptomatic. However, if the diverticula contain ectopic gastric mucosa, the acid can produce bleeding in the ileum. A narrow-necked Meckel's diverticulum can obstruct and can mimic appendicitis. On rare occasions, the diverticulum can become a lead point for intussusception, thus causing small-bowel obstruction.

Indications for surgery for a Meckel's diverticulum include hemorrhage, obstruction, and perforation.

Crohn's Disease

Crohn's disease, an inflammatory disease of the small intestine of unknown origin, occasionally requires surgical therapy. Patients with Crohn's disease most frequently present with abdominal pain, which can mimic appendicitis. Most cases of Crohn's disease are treated medically with corticosteroids.

PEARL: Many complications of Crohn's disease require surgical therapy. The following are such complications:

- Obstruction
- Perforation
- Fistula (Note that fistulas beginning in the small bowel or colon may communicate with the bowel, bladder, vagina, or skin.)
- Hemorrhage
- Intractable pain (failure of medication)

Patients requiring surgery for complications of Crohn's disease frequently need a bowel resection.

**Table 15–2. COMPARISON OF CROHN'S
DISEASE AND ULCERATIVE COLITIS**

Parameter	Crohn's Disease	Ulcerative Colitis
Etiology	Unknown	Unknown
Pathology	Transmural	Mucosal
Disease pattern	Small bowel and/or colon	Colon
Therapy	Corticosteroids	Corticosteroids and/or sulfasalazine
Presentation	Abdominal pain	Rectal bleeding
Cancer risk	Low	High
Systemic (non-GI) manifestations	Unusual	Common

Some patients need numerous operations during their
lifetime. If left with inadequate length of small bowel,
patients may end up with **short-bowel syndrome,**
which is characterized by malnutrition and fluid and
electrolyte problems.

Crohn's disease has some similarities to and differences from ulcerative colitis (Table 15–2). Ulcerative
colitis is discussed in detail in Chapter 16.

16
CHAPTER

Colon

COLON CANCER

The colon prepares waste products of digestion for elimination. With water absorption, liquid stool in the right colon is converted to solid stool in the sigmoid colon. This change in fecal consistency has clinical relevance in the understanding of the clinical presentation of colon cancer.

Colon cancer is common in both men and women. Left-sided (rectosigmoid) cancers are most common. Cancers in the transverse colon are unusual. Because stool in the left colon is solid, when a cancer impedes the lumen, the patient has obstructive symptoms (discomfort, constipation). Conversely, with liquid stool proximally, cancers of the right colon do not obstruct. Patients with right-sided colon cancers present with guaiac-positive stool and anemia.

Pathogenesis

Most authorities believe in the **adenoma-carcinoma sequence.** This means that most colon cancers begin as adenomatous polyps. The most exaggerated example of this is in patients with familial or multiple polyposis syndrome. Such patients are at extraordinarily high risk for the development of colon cancer. Therefore, most patients with familial polyposis have a total colectomy before adulthood.

Because many polyps bleed mildly, adult patients with occult fecal blood are screened with flexible colonoscopy. Patients with a history of colon polyps or a family history of colon cancer are also subjected to periodic colonoscopy. Colonoscopy allows detection of colon cancer at early stages so that the tumors may be amenable to surgical cure.

Colon cancer is classified by depth of penetration of the tumor and by nodal status (Table 16–1). This classification also gives us prognostic information.

Treatment and Prognosis

Operations designed for colon cancer are intended to resect both the tumor and the regional nodal basin (Table 16–2). The regional nodes are near the blood vessels in the mesocolon. The cancer operation also gives us prognostic (staging) information. There are no large prospective studies comparing outcomes after radical resection versus a more conservative or segmental resection.

CONTROVERSY: It is not known whether a wide nodal resection increases cure rates.

Five-year survival rates after surgical resection are listed in Table 16–1.

Patients with Duke's B2 and C lesions probably benefit from chemotherapy with 5-fluorouracil and levamisole. Radiation therapy may be used preoperatively to

Table 16–1. DUKE'S CLASSIFICATION OF COLORECTAL CANCER

Class	Depth	5-Year Survival Rate
A	Limited to muscularis	90%
B1	Through muscularis	70%
B2	Through muscularis to serosa	50%
C	Any depth with positive nodes	30–40%
D	Distal metastasis	<20%

Table 16–2. TYPES OF OPERATION FOR COLON CANCER

Tumor Location	Procedure
Right colon	Right hemicolectomy
Transverse colon	Transverse colectomy
Descending colon	Left hemicolectomy
Sigmoid colon	Sigmoid colectomy
Upper rectum	Anterior rectosigmoid resection
Lower rectum	Abdominal-perineal resection of rectum and anus

shrink rectal cancers and to limit long-term pelvic recurrences. In proximal (nonrectal) colon cancer, radiation therapy is used for advanced local spread.

DIVERTICULAR DISEASE

Diverticula in the colon are acquired *false* diverticula. True diverticulae have all bowel layers (e.g., Meckel's diverticulum). The presence of colonic diverticula is called **diverticulosis.**

Colonic diverticula are herniations of mucosa through muscularis and thus have only mucosal and serosal layers (and are prone to perforation). These diverticula are associated with a Western (low-fiber) diet. More than 50% of adults over the age of 50 in the United States have colonic diverticula.

Location of Diverticula

Colonic diverticula are most common in the sigmoid colon. Progression to microperforation results in acute infection due to colonic bacteria leaking from the perforation. This process usually seals, resulting in a diverticular abscess or infection of the colon wall and pericolonic fat. **PEARL: Sigmoid diverticulitis presents as *"left-sided appendicitis,"* with left lower quadrant pain, fever, and leukocytosis.**

Treatment Considerations

The following are important points to consider in treatment of diverticular disease:

- Most patients respond to gut rest plus IV antibiotics. Thus the initial treatment of sigmoid diverticulitis is *medical.*
- If the patient does not improve by 48 hours following initiation of medical treatment (with lowered temperature, decrease in white blood cells [WBCs], and resolution of pain), then surgery may be required.
- A less common indication for surgery with sigmoid diverticulitis is free perforation (unsealed) with peritonitis—a surgical emergency.
- Most cases of sigmoid diverticulitis requiring surgery are treated with sigmoid colectomy plus colostomy.
- In the worst cases (those with septic shock or the medically unfit patient), only a diverting colostomy is done; this diverts the fecal stream away from the infection. With only a diverting colostomy, however, one must rely on IV antibiotics to treat the remaining infected sigmoid. One can see why removing the infected organ is preferable.
- A patient who has had two hospital admissions for sigmoid diverticulitis (treated medically) is at high risk for further attack of life-threatening sepsis. Therefore, elective sigmoid colectomy with primary anastomosis is recommended.
- Left-sided *tics* (diverticula) don't usually bleed. Diverticula of the right colon are more prone to hemorrhage.

A second disorder of the colon associated with aging is **vascular ectasia,** which consists of enlarged microvessels of the submucosa. Ectasias are most common in the cecum and right colon. Diverticula and vascular ectasias are the most common causes of massive lower GI bleeding in adults (see Chapter 18).

ULCERATIVE COLITIS

Ulcerative colitis is an inflammatory disease of the colonic mucosa of unknown cause. Patients present with significant red rectal bleeding. The rectum is never spared; therefore, the *activity* of disease may be gauged by annual flexible sigmoidoscopy.

The extent of involvement of the proximal colon varies. Ulcerative proctitis with normal ascending transverse, descending, and sigmoid colon is a mild form of ulcerative colitis.

PEARL: Patients with active ulcerative colitis for 10 years have a 3% incidence of colon cancer. This percentage rises 2 to 3% per year thereafter. To avoid this, these patients have colon biopsies annually. The development of severe dysplasia is an indication for panproctocolectomy. Note the comparison between ulcerative colitis and Crohn's disease in Chapter 15.

When operating for ulcerative colitis (because of massive hemorrhage, failure of medical therapy, or malignancy), the entire colon, rectum, and rectal mucosa to the anus must be removed. Table 16–3 shows reconstruction options and their advantages and disadvantages.

Table 16–3. ADVANTAGES AND DISADVANTAGES OF RECONSTRUCTION OPTIONS FOR ULCERATIVE COLITIS

Procedure	Advantages	Disadvantages
Standard Brooke ileostomy*	Surgically simple, few complications	Patient wears permanent bag.
Continent ileostomy*	No constant fecal leakage	Patient must periodically intubate and drain.
Ileoanal pull-through[†]	Maintains anal sphincter, no "ostomy"	Patients have 4–10 bowel movements daily; sometimes there is nocturnal leakage.

*Older patients (>50 years) may wish to avoid reliving "potty training" and choose an ileostomy.
[†]In general, younger patients (<50 years) requiring total colectomy for ulcerative colitis should be offered an ileoanal pull-through.

SIGMOID VOLVULUS

As we age, our colons elongate. For example, a redundant sigmoid colon that revolves around its mesocolonic axis results in a closed-loop colonic obstruction and the potential for colonic necrosis.

Sigmoid volvulus has a classic plain x-ray appearance with massively dilated colon flipped toward the right upper quadrant (Fig. 16–1). This condition is an emer-

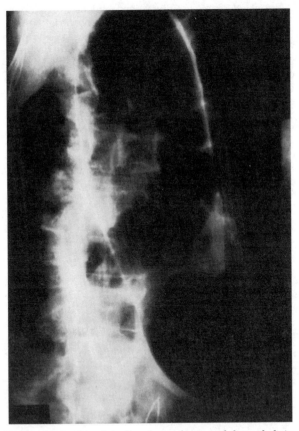

Figure 16–1. This plain film shows the typical distended sigmoid colon filling most of the abdomen in a sigmoid volvulus.

gency and treatment is with flexible or rigid sigmoid-oscopy, which untwists and decompresses the twisted colon. A flexible rectal tube is placed to prevent immediate revolvulus. The patient is later taken for elective sigmoid colectomy, if medically fit for surgery.

BOWEL PREPARATION
FOR ELECTIVE COLECTOMY

Before elective (nonobstructed) colectomy, a bowel "prep" is needed, to decrease colonic bacterial counts. Feces are collections of debris and bacteria. The **prep** must eliminate all solid fecal matter. The most common preps are liters of oral lavage fluid (like polyethylene glycol electrolyte solution [GoLYTELY]), which the patient drinks. Other options are oral citrate of magnesium combined with saline enemas. To decrease bacterial counts even more, poorly absorbed oral antibiotics such as neomycin and erythromycin base may be added.

With a clean, prepped colon, anastomoses can be done with low infection and leak rates. Colonic anastomoses may be hand-sewn (sutured) or stapled using any of a variety of stapling instruments.

17
CHAPTER

Anorectum

Anorectal complaints are very common in office practice. Common complaints include:

- Pain
- Rectal bleeding
- Fecal soiling of underwear

COMMON ANORECTAL PROBLEMS

The most common anorectal disorder is **hemorrhoids.**

Internal hemorrhoids are enlarged versions of normal venous cushions within the lower rectum. **PEARL: Contrary to what is seen on television commercials, internal hemorrhoids generally do not cause pain. The most common problem caused by internal hemorrhoids is red rectal bleeding.** Bleeding from internal hemorrhoids occurs at the end of a bowel movement and stains the toilet water and toilet tissue red. The treatment of internal hemorrhoids based on size is shown in Table 17–1.

External hemorrhoids occur distal to the dentate line. A thrombosed external hemorrhoid presents as a painful, tender, purple-black, perianal lump.

Fissures are tears in the skin and anal mucosa. These are usually in the posterior midline and present with pain particularly with defecation.

Perirectal abscesses occur in the subcutaneous fat adjacent to the anus. They frequently extend proximally

Table 17–1. TREATMENT OF INTERNAL HEMORRHOIDS BASED ON SIZE

Degree	Definition	Treatment
First	Hemorrhoid to the dentate line	Diet and defecatory modification
Second	Outside anal canal with bowel movement (self-reducing)	Rubber banding or injection therapy
Third	Outside anal canal with bowel movement (requiring digital reduction)	As above or hemorrhoidectomy
Fourth	Incarcerated outside anal canal	Hemorrhoidectomy

along the outer rectal wall and occasionally above the levator muscles. These abscesses are painful, particularly when the patient is sitting. The perirectal abscess is fluctuant to the palpating finger, and the skin over the abscess is red.

Fistula-in-ano is a fistula that connects the rectal lumen with the skin (bypassing the sphincter mechanisms). Thus, a patient with a fistula-in-ano presents with fecal soiling of underwear.

Tumors of the rectum are not uncommon. For example:

- **Villous adenomas** are sessile, soft, raised masses. The larger the villous adenoma, the greater the chance of its harboring a malignancy.
- **Adenocarcinomas** commonly occur in the rectum. Small tumors may be treated with local resection through an operating proctoscope. Larger cancers require colorectal resection.

Some patients insist that they are too tender to undergo digital rectal examination. In this case, they should be scheduled for an examination under anesthesia (EUA). EUA includes both digital examination and anoscopy. **PEARL: Remember that patients with squamous cell carcinoma of the anus can present with anal pain and tenderness. Therefore, EUA should not be deferred for weeks or months.**

Table 17–2. TREATMENT OF COMMON ANORECTAL PROBLEMS

Condition	Symptom	Treatment
Thrombosed external hemorrhoid	Pain (tender purple-black mass)	Hemorrhoidectomy under local or incision and evacuation of clot
Fissure	Pain (posterior midline)	Lateral internal sphincterotomy
Perirectal abscess	Pain	Incision and drainage
Fistula-in-ano	Fecal soiling of underwear	Fistulotomy

Treatment

Many anorectal problems can be treated in the office. Severe cases are treated in the operating room. See Table 17–2 for the various treatment methods for common anorectal problems.

For a discussion of colorectal cancer, see Chapter 16.

18

Acute Gastrointestinal Bleeding

Gastrointestinal (GI) bleeding is usually classified according to the clinical presentation. Thus, patients with hematemesis are classified as upper GI bleeders, and patients with melena (black, tarry stools) or hematochezia (red, rectal bleeding) are classified as lower GI bleeders. This classification is somewhat artificial because most patients with melena actually have a source proximal to the ligament of Treitz.

Upper and lower GI bleeding have certain things in common. **PEARL: First, more than 70% of cases stop bleeding spontaneously.** Also, the approach to both upper and lower GI bleeding is similar, consisting of three phases:

- Resuscitation
- Evaluation
- Treatment

RESUSCITATION

Resuscitation involves restoration of the intravascular volume by administration of crystalloid (balanced salt solution). The following steps are necessary for successful resuscitation:

- The patient is typed and cross-matched in case blood transfusion becomes necessary. It is preferable to have two large-bore IV lines to keep up with fluid and blood requirements.
- A baseline hemoglobin is obtained, but it is understood that it will be falsely high owing to hemoconcentration. Postresuscitation hemoglobin levels reflect true blood volume loss.
- A Foley catheter is placed to monitor the success of resuscitation (indirect measure of renal perfusion).
- If the patient is hypotensive, IV fluid resuscitation proceeds with IVs "wide open."
- In normotensive patients, resolution of compensatory tachycardia and establishment of acceptable urine output are guides to successful resuscitation.

EVALUATION

The evaluation phase differs in approach, depending on whether an upper or lower source is expected. Whether GI bleeding is from an upper or a lower source, the patient history is important. Many diseases causing GI bleeding (e.g., peptic ulcer and esophageal varices) are recurrent or persistent disorders. In addition, blood dyscrasias or coagulopathies may be suggested by history or physical examination.

Upper GI Bleeding

With an upper GI source, endoscopic examination may be successful despite ongoing bleeding. This is because the esophagus, stomach, and duodenum may be cleared with lavage and suction. The large diameter of the stomach allows for endoscope mobility and visualization.

Causes

- Peptic ulcer
- Erosive gastritis
- Esophageal varices
- Mallory-Weiss tear

Lower GI Bleeding

With active lower GI bleeding, segments of colon fill with blood and are difficult to clear. The narrow lumen full of blood precludes visualization via colonoscopy.

Therefore, unless the patient has stopped bleeding, tagged red blood cell (RBC) nuclear scan or selective mesenteric angiograms are commonly needed to establish the bleeding site. If the lower GI bleed stops, a bowel prep and colonoscopy are possible.

Causes

- Colonic diverticula
- Vascular ectasias of the colon
- Ulcerative colitis (less common)

Table 18–1 lists probable sources of lower GI bleeding.

Common Causes of Bleeding

Mallory-Weiss tears are mucosal (nontransmural) tears in the gastric mucosa just beyond the gastroesophageal junction. They are associated with severe vomiting and retching. These lesions usually bleed for less than 24 hours and resolve spontaneously.

Esophageal varices are dilated veins in the lower esophagus that connect the portal to the systemic venous circulation. They are due to portal hypertension,

Table 18–1. LOWER GI BLEEDING PATTERN AND PROBABLE SOURCE

Pattern	Probable Source
Melena	Stomach or duodenum
Mahogany stool	Small bowel or right colon
Red blood stool	Colon
Red toilet water with brown stool	Hemorrhoids

which in turn is due to cirrhosis of the liver. The most common therapy for bleeding esophageal varices is endoscopic therapy, either injection sclerotherapy or rubber banding. If endoscopic therapy cannot be performed because of unavailability or massive hemorrhage, placement of an esophageal balloon catheter (Sengstaken-Blakemore or Minnesota tube) may be lifesaving (Fig. 18–1). Portal venous decompression via operative portosystemic shunting or transvenous intrahepatic portosystemic shunting (TIPs) procedures are additional options.

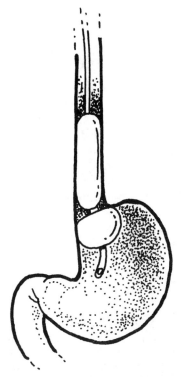

Figure 18–1. Correct placement of a Sengstaken-Blakemore tube. Note position of both the gastric and the esophageal balloons.

Note that cancers are not among the sources of bleeding. **PEARL: Esophageal, gastric, and colon cancers generally do not cause massive GI bleeding.** Instead, they cause occult bleeding detected on stool guaiac exams. Chronic occult bleeding results in microcytic, iron deficiency anemia.

Note also that internal hemorrhoids are not listed among the causes of bleeding. Although hemorrhoids frequently cause significant red rectal bleeding, the pattern should be readily discernible by history. Specifically, internal hemorrhoids cause bright red staining of toilet water and toilet tissue. The stool in these cases is normal brown in color and not mixed with blood.

Gastritis, peptic ulcer, and colonic lesions are discussed elsewhere in this book.

TREATMENT

The treatment phase of acute GI bleeding depends on the cause of the bleed and the urgency of the situation. As noted, most cases stop bleeding spontaneously, thus allowing for elective therapy.

Surgery

Indications

- Massive, unrelenting (active) bleeding
- Cases requiring 5 or more units of blood
- Patients who re-bleed during hospitalization
- Duodenal ulcers with a visible vessel
- Patients readmitted for second bleed

Bleeding Ulcers

Bleeding peptic ulcers requiring surgery are treated differently based on site. Bleeding duodenal ulcers are treated with suture ligation (oversewing) of the bleeding vessel. An anti-ulcer operation (see Chapter 12) may be added if the patient is otherwise healthy (and stable). Bleeding gastric ulcers are frequently treated with partial gastrectomy (to include ulcer resection).

Bleeding colonic lesions requiring surgery are treated with segmental colectomy. **PEARL: Frequently, it is difficult to precisely localize the site of a lower GI bleed.** If the bleed is isolated to the colon but the precise locale cannot be determined, a subtotal colectomy with ileorectal anastomosis may be performed.

Endoscopic Therapy

Endoscopic therapy is frequently used in lieu of surgery. Lasers, electrocautery, and heater probes may stop bleeding in the stomach, duodenum, and colon. In some circumstances, embolic therapy via angiographically guided catheter may be used.

CONTROVERSY: Embolic therapy may be unsuccessful in upper GI bleeding owing to the multiple arterial arcades. In the colon, embolic therapy brings the risk of bowel wall necrosis.

19
CHAPTER

Hernias

TYPES AND ANATOMY OF HERNIAS

Inguinal (groin) hernias are among the most common disorders seen by the general surgeon. Inguinal hernia repair is the most common operation performed by general surgeons. These hernias are more common in men.

The three types of groin hernias are indirect, direct, and femoral.

- **Indirect hernias** occur through the deep ring, which is a natural defect in the floor of the inguinal canal. These hernias include a peritoneal sac (a patent processus vaginalis).
- **Direct hernias** occur through acquired defects in the floor (transversalis fascia). They are thought to be occupational (heavy lifting) or caused by repeated "wear and tear." Some believe that repeated straining to urinate or defecate past an obstruction (enlarged prostate or rectal tumor) contributes to hernia development in some patients. A careful review of these aspects of the patient's history helps to determine whether colonic or prostatic evaluations are needed before hernia repair.

Another way to define direct and indirect hernias is in relation to the inferior epigastric vessels. Indirect hernias occur lateral to these vessels. Direct hernias occur medial to the vessels (Fig. 19–1).

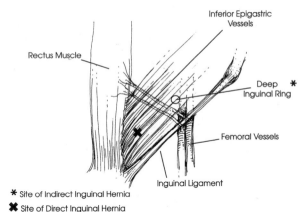

Figure 19–1. Anatomy of the groin. X demonstrates site of direct hernias, through floor of inguinal canal, medial to epigastric vessels.

Note that direct hernias occur through an area called **Hasselbach's triangle.** The triangle is made of the lateral edge of the rectus medially, the inguinal ligament laterally, and the epigastric vessels superiorly.

- **Femoral hernias** occur through the femoral canal (Fig. 19–2). **PEARL: The mnemonic for femoral anatomy is NAVEL: femoral *nerve,* femoral *artery,* femoral *vein, empty* space, *ligament.*** Femoral hernias occur through this empty space.

Sliding hernias (direct, indirect, or femoral) are hernias in which an internal organ (such as bowel or bladder) forms one wall of the contents of the hernia. In other words, the peritoneal sac may exist for 270 degrees rather than 360 degrees of the circumference. **PEARL: It is important to avoid injury to viscera during repair of a sliding hernia.**

The anatomy of hernias must be understood to appreciate the logic of various hernia repairs. For example, if the inguinal canal is thought of in three dimensions, it has a floor, a roof, a medial wall, and a lateral wall (Fig. 19–3*A* and *B*).

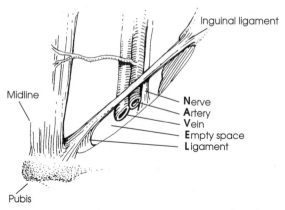

Figure 19–2. Anatomy of femoral vessels at the inguinal level.

- The **roof** is the fascia of the external oblique muscle.
- The **floor** is made up of transversalis fascia.
- The **medial wall** of the canal is the "conjoined tendon." (This is not really a tendon but is the fused fascia of the internal oblique and transversalis muscles.)
- The **lateral wall** of the canal is the shelving edge of the inguinal ligament.

The deepest border of the shelving edge is the ileopubic tract. Hernias occur through the floor of the inguinal canal. They therefore occur through defects in the transversalis fascia. Repairs must reconstitute the transversalis fascia. The spermatic cord (vas deferens and testicular vessels) passes from intra-abdominal up through the deep (internal) inguinal ring into the inguinal canal, exiting at the external ring.

HERNIA REPAIRS

Hernias are repaired both to eliminate associated discomfort and to prevent serious complications.

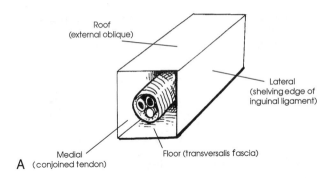

Inguinal Canal

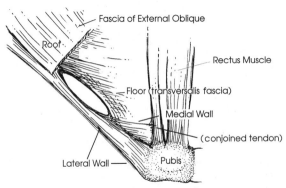

Figure 19–3. (*A*) Schematic drawing of left inguinal canal in three dimensions as viewed from the patient's feet toward the head. (*B*) Anatomy of the right inguinal canal with the "roof" (exterior oblique fascia) removed.

Types

Bassini

Indirect hernias were traditionally corrected with a Bassini repair, described by Eduardo Bassini more than 90 years ago. With this repair, the peritoneal hernial sac (always present with an indirect hernia) is ligated at the deep ring level. (This is known as "high ligation.") The distal sac is amputated. Finally, the conjoined tendon medially is sutured to the ileopubic tract laterally, thus eliminating the defect (which is a dilated deep ring).

McVay

Direct hernias have traditionally been repaired with a McVay repair, described by Chester McVay over 40 years ago. With this repair, the conjoined tendon medially is sutured to Cooper's ligament inferolaterally. Finally, the proximal conjoined tendon is brought to the ileopubic tract laterally (as in the Bassini repair). This reconstitutes the floor of the inguinal canal. **PEARL: A McVay repair also closes the femoral empty space and thus can be used to repair femoral hernias.**

Shouldice

In a Shouldice repair, the transversalis fascia (floor of the inguinal canal) is incised and closed by overlapping the medial and lateral segments with two running suture lines. Thus, the weakened transversalis is strengthened by doubling its thickness (via overlap).

Tension-Free

During the 1990s, "tension-free" prosthetic repairs became very popular. With these repairs, prosthetic patch (polypropylene or Gore-Tex) is laid over the floor of the inguinal canal and sutured to Cooper's ligament inferolaterally, to the ileopubic tract laterally, and to the conjoined tendon medially. The theoretical advantage is that the repair avoids the tension sometimes required to pull native tissues together. At many centers, the tension-free prosthetic repair has replaced Bassini and McVay repairs.

Laparoscopic

In the past 6 or 7 years, laparoscopic repair has been introduced (see Chapter 7). With laparoscopic repair, a prosthetic is introduced intra-abdominally or preperitoneally and stapled to the deep surface of the transversalis fascia, thus covering the hernia defect.

Advantages of laparoscopic hernia repair are less pain and quicker recovery.

Disadvantages are that more general anesthetic is needed and it is an expensive procedure.

Conventional inguinal hernia repairs (nonlaparoscopic) can be performed with local, spinal, or epidural anesthesia. Laparoscopic repairs require a general anesthetic.

CONTROVERSY: It is not clear whether laparoscopic hernia repair offers any significant advantage over conventional repair.

Self-Reduction and Incarceration

Many hernias bulge out with standing or exercise and self-reduce when the patient lies down. Sometimes a hernia does not spontaneously reduce and requires manual reduction. **PEARL: When a hernia cannot be reduced (contents are trapped in the hernia), it is said to be "incarcerated."** An **incarcerated hernia** is a surgical emergency. If left alone, an incarcerated hernia may go on to strangulate. A **strangulated hernia** occurs when the contents of the hernia have lost their blood supply. This condition can cause death due to sepsis, particularly if bowel is trapped in the hernia. Thus, elective repairs are performed both to minimize discomfort and to prevent life-threatening complications.

Recurrence

About 3 to 10% of hernias recur after being repaired, sometimes years later. Repairing recurrent hernias is more difficult than de novo hernia repair. This is due to scarring, which fuses normally distinct fascial layers. This fusing increases the complication rate, particularly injury to the ileoinguinal nerve. Because a laparoscopic repair avoids the scarred inguinal canal (by working beneath it), some authorities feel that a laparoscopic approach is preferred for repair of recurrent hernias.

Complications

As with any operation, surgeons strive to avoid post-operative complications resulting from hernia repair. Complications include the following:

- Nerve injury (1 to 2%)
- Urinary retention (10%)
- Recurrent hernia (3 to 10%)
- Visceral injury (rare)

NONINGUINAL HERNIAS

Ventral hernias are usually hernias in the midline of the abdomen. The most common is **epigastric** hernia. If a ventral hernia is in an old incision, it is more properly called an **incisional** hernia. **Umbilical hernias** are relatively common. The concept of repair of any of these hernias is closure of the fascial defect. If the fascial defect is large (e.g., >4 cm wide), most surgeons consider a repair with prosthetic mesh.

3
PART

ICU/Trauma

20
CHAPTER

Initial Assessment of the Trauma Patient

OVERVIEW

Trauma is a leading cause of morbidity and mortality, particularly among young adults. The cost in health care dollars expended on trauma patients is enormous. Obviously, prevention is the key to controlling this epidemic. Until that happens, we must be prepared to manage trauma patients.

The initial evaluation and assessment of trauma patients have been standardized by the American College of Surgeons into a text and course called *Advanced Trauma Life Support* (ATLS). This is an organized, consistent approach that optimizes the chances for recognition of injuries and provides for optimal resuscitation and final outcome. This chapter is a condensation of the ATLS text and focuses on the initial evaluation and assessment of trauma patients. Students of surgery interested in further reading should refer to the full text.

Time Distribution of Deaths from Trauma

Death from trauma has a trimodal distribution:

- The first peak occurs seconds to minutes after injury and, because of the severity of the injuries, these trauma patients are usually dead at the scene. Such injuries include massive head and high spinal cord injuries and exsanguination due to lacerations/tears of the heart, aorta, or other major vessels.
- The second peak (termed the golden hour) occurs minutes to hours after trauma. ATLS is geared toward saving the lives of these patients during this time period.
- The third peak occurs days to weeks after injury. Deaths during this time period are primarily due to sepsis and organ failure.

Phases of Assessment

The overall assessment of trauma patients is divided into three parts or phases:

1. Primary survey: ABCs
2. Resuscitation phase
3. Secondary survey

The final phase in dealing with the trauma patient is the definitive care phase. Subsequent chapters deal with specific types of injuries and their management.

PRIMARY SURVEY: ABCs

The ABCs of trauma are modified somewhat from those of ACLS. They are actually ABCDE and take into consideration several trauma-specific issues. The ABCs of trauma include the following:

Airway maintenance with cervical spine control
Breathing and ventilation
Circulation and hemorrhage control
Disability—Neurologic status
Exposure—Completely undress the patient

This list presents the initial priorities that should be followed in order of importance. Usually, these survey areas are addressed simultaneously by various members of the trauma team. However, the clinician in charge must ensure that airway management is always the top priority.

Airway Maintenance with Cervical Spine Control

All trauma patients, regardless of the degree of injury, require an immediate assessment of airway patency. **PEARL: The quickest way of ensuring a patent, working airway (as well as a conscious, mentally alert patient) is by getting an appropriate verbal response after asking a patient how he or she is doing.** The following are steps in this assessment process:

- Look, listen, and feel to assess the airway.
- Look for agitation (hypoxia), obtundation (hypercarbia), and cyanosis.
- Listen for abnormal sounds (gurgling, snoring, hoarseness) that suggest airway compromise.
- Feel for airway movement during expiration.

Manual Maneuvers

PEARL: In trauma, all patients are considered to have a cervical spinal cord injury and are treated accordingly until it has been proven that no such injury exists. Maintain neck immobilization throughout initial management. Therefore, all attempts to maintain or establish airway patency must be done while maintaining cervical spine stability (in-line traction), usually in a cervical collar (or "C collar"). Flexion or extension of the neck is never performed, and maneuvers such as the chin lift and jaw thrust to establish airway patency are initially relied on.

The removal of foreign debris, blood, or secretions from the airway also takes place at this point. In the absence of maxillofacial trauma, an oropharyngeal airway (curved, plastic device that keeps tongue up) or nasopharyngeal airway (curved, plastic tube inserted into nose) may be placed to help maintain airway patency in a patient who is breathing spontaneously.

Intubation and Cricothyroidotomy

PEARL: If the chin lift and jaw thrust fail to establish a patent airway or if the patient is unresponsive, advanced airway intervention with oral endotracheal or nasotracheal intubation is required. Oral endotracheal intubation is more commonly practiced because it is easier, quicker, and more reliable than nasotracheal intubation. It must be performed without extending the patient's neck (because cervical spine injury has not yet been ruled out) and while maintaining in-line neck immobilization. If the patient is breathing spontaneously and has no evidence of maxillofacial trauma, nasotracheal intubation is another option.

If endotracheal intubation fails (e.g., cords are not visible owing to blood or secretions, distorted anatomy, or edema from injury) or is contraindicated because of severe maxillofacial or laryngeal injury, surgical airway intervention via a cricothyroidotomy is required.

Cricothyroidotomy involves making an incision (with a scalpel) over the cricothyroid membrane. After the membrane is incised, a tracheostomy or endotracheal tube is inserted directly into the trachea. In experienced hands, this procedure takes less than 1 minute. For a patient with a marginal airway where endotracheal intubation is initially attempted but thought to be difficult, it is advisable to be prepared (e.g., neck prepped and anesthetized, scalpel in hand) to perform a cricothyroidotomy. (In children under 12 years, a needle cricothyroidotomy is preferred.)

Breathing and Ventilation

Once an airway is established, ventilation is initially assessed by observing a patient's chest rise and fall with inspiration and expiration. Auscultation of the chest is performed to assure equal breath sounds bilaterally. Ventilation is aided by applying a bag-valve device attached to a face mask or endotracheal tube. Ensure adequate oxygenation by providing supplemental oxygen (100% oxygen during early stages of ventilation), especially if the patient required intubation.

PEARL: Three life-threatening ventilatory conditions that must be recognized and treated in the primary survey

are tension pneumothorax, open pneumothorax, and flail chest with pulmonary contusion.

Tension Pneumothorax

Patients with tension pneumothorax classically present with markedly decreased or absent breath sounds over one side of the chest, distended neck veins and hypotension. The pathophysiology involves lung injury (rib fracture and subsequent lung laceration) with subsequent accumulation of air under pressure in the pleural space. As the pressure builds, the lung is compressed and the mediastinum is shifted toward the other side. The resulting kinking of the superior and inferior vena cava causes diminished venous return to the heart, a decreased cardiac output, and hypotension. The backup of blood in the superior vena cava results in neck vein distention. Classically, the mediastinal shift can progress to deviate the trachea to the other side, but this is a late and rarely seen sign.

If there is a diagnosis or suspicion of tension pneumothorax, treatment must be initiated quickly and should not be delayed pending x-ray confirmation.

Initial treatment of tension pneumothorax consists of thrusting a large-bore needle (preferably 14-gauge) into the second interspace (opposite the angle of Louis) in the midclavicular line of the affected side of the chest (needle decompression). If tension pneumothorax is present, a whoosh of air comes from the catheter, thus confirming the diagnosis. The release of the intrapleural air and pressure restores ventilation and reverses hypotension. Finally, inserting a chest tube offers continued and definitive management.

Open Pneumothorax

Blunt or penetrating trauma can cause an open pneumothorax (communication through the chest wall and into the pleural space). If the open defect is sufficiently large, negative intrapleural pressure (with respiratory effort) preferentially pulls air through the defect rather than through the trachea, resulting in the classic sucking chest wound. With this type of trauma the underlying lung is usually (though not always) injured.

Management of open pneumothorax consists of placing an occlusive dressing over the opening and either taping it on three of four sides (thus creating a valve-like effect to allow intrapleural air out but not in) or taping it on all sides and placing a chest tube at a remote site to prevent development of a tension pneumothorax. The chest wall defect usually requires surgical closure during the definitive treatment phase.

Flail Chest

Flail chest with pulmonary contusion results from severe blunt chest trauma. Typically, multiple rib fractures in more than one location create a segment of chest wall that no longer moves in continuity with the rest of the chest. This alteration in pulmonary mechanics impairs ventilation and, along with the even more significant underlying pulmonary contusion, results in hypoxemia.

Management of flail chest usually requires intubation and mechanical ventilation with positive pressure to achieve lung expansion.

Circulation and Hemorrhage Control

This component of the primary survey is designed to rapidly (e.g., in seconds) assess the injured patient's hemodynamic status. **PEARL: During the primary survey, circulation is assessed by checking three parameters: mental status, skin color, and hemodynamic status (heart rate and blood pressure).**

- Mental status. Patients who have lost large volumes of blood (>40–50% blood volume) are usually unconscious as a result of inadequate cerebral blood flow. A fully conscious patient obviously has adequate cerebral perfusion, although this hardly means the patient is out of trouble.
- Skin color. Pale (usually ashen gray or white) rather than pink skin is a sign of significant blood loss. This change in skin color is caused by both blood loss and peripheral vasoconstriction (a response to hypovolemia). Another quick way of assessing this vasoconstrictive response is to perform

a capillary blanch test by pressing the patient's fingernail bed and observing how quickly it pinks up when released. An interval of more than 2 seconds is considered abnormal and, during trauma, is usually a sign of significant blood loss.

- Hemodynamic status. The pulse is assessed both for its rate and fullness. **PEARL: Hemodynamic instability, defined as HR greater than 100 or systolic blood pressure less than 90, is considered due to blood loss until proven otherwise** (see Chapter 24, section on Hypovolemic and Hemorrhagic Shock).

Obvious external bleeding must be recognized and controlled at this time by direct pressure over the bleeding area or by application of a splint to a fractured extremity. Use of hemostats to control bleeding is dangerous because of poor visualization and the likelihood of causing additional vascular or nerve injury. Tourniquets are also ill advised.

Pericardial Tamponade

One life-threatening complication that must be diagnosed quickly in the trauma patient at this point is **pericardial tamponade. PEARL: The classic triad (Beck's triad) of hypotension, distended neck veins, and muffled heart sounds is present in fewer than half of patients who are found to have pericardial tamponade.** Therefore, one must maintain a high level of suspicion in any patient with a precordial penetrating injury and *any one* of the above-mentioned signs. (The precordial area extends from the suprasternal notch to the xiphoid and from nipple to nipple on the anterior and posterior chest.)

The pathophysiology of pericardial tamponade involves a cardiac injury with leakage of blood into the pericardial sac. This sac normally contains about 10 to 20 mL of fluid. The addition of as little as 20 to 50 mL of blood can impair venous filling of the ventricles. As a result, cardiac output is markedly depressed, resulting in hypotension. Distended neck veins result from impaired emptying of the superior and inferior vena cava into the heart, and the resulting increased venous pressure transmitted up the neck veins.

PEARL: Diagnosis and initial management of pericardial tamponade consist of subxiphoid pericardiocentesis or pericardial window.

In **subxiphoid pericardiocentesis,** a long needle is passed beneath the xiphoid in the direction of the heart's apex to tap into and remove some of the pericardial blood. Removal of even small amounts of blood can have dramatic effects in improving hemodynamic status and providing enough time to transport the patient to the operating room for definitive care.

CONTROVERSY: Because of the difficulty in performing subxiphoid pericardiocentesis and its often nondefinitive results, many trauma surgeons prefer to perform a definitive subxiphoid pericardial window (Trinkle procedure) in the operating room.

In the **pericardial window** procedure, an incision is made above and below the xiphoid and an ample-sized area of pericardium at the base of the heart is exposed and incised. If blood is encountered, definitive cardiac exploration and repair are undertaken via a median sternotomy or anterolateral thoracotomy incision. If clear fluid is found, then tamponade is definitively ruled out and evaluation of the patient, as needed, continues in the operating room. Bedside ultrasound, now available in many emergency rooms, is assuming a growing role in the diagnosis of pericardial tamponade.

Disability—Neurologic Status

Because of the high morbidity associated with neurologic injuries, a rapid assessment of level of consciousness and pupillary function is conducted. In an abridged form of the Glasgow Coma Scale, level of consciousness is assigned to one of four categories, based on the acronym AVPU:

A—**A**lert
V—Responds to **v**erbal stimuli
P—Responds to **p**ainful stimuli
U—**U**nresponsive

Pupillary size and reactivity to light are also checked during the initial assessment. Abnormalities in level of consciousness or pupillary reactivity can be signs of intracranial injury or decreased cerebral oxygenation and perfusion.

Exposure—Completely Undress the Patient

The final part of the primary survey is to completely undress the patient to facilitate a thorough visual examination. This usually takes place early in the primary survey as personnel remove or cut away all clothes and jewelry.

RESUSCITATION

During the resuscitation phase, a number of steps are accomplished to provide support to the injured patient and begin fluid resuscitation. **PEARL: The resuscitation phase consists of providing supplemental oxygen, beginning fluid resuscitation with 2 liters lactated Ringer's solution via two large-bore peripheral IVs, electrocardiogram (ECG) monitoring, nasogastric tube and Foley insertion, and lab evaluation.**

Oxygen

All patients get supplemental oxygen, initially either in the form of a 100% reservoir face mask or 100% oxygen via a ventilator if the patient is intubated. Pulse oximetry is used to determine the adequacy of oxygenation (although pulse oximetry may be unreliable in a hypothermic and poorly perfused patient).

Fluid Resuscitation

IV Lines

Fluid resuscitation begins with the placement of two large-bore (16-gauge or larger) IV lines, usually placed in the antecubital fossa of each arm. Large-bore peripheral IVs are much more effective for resuscitation than central lines because resistance to flow is inversely related to the catheter's radius (to the fourth degree) and directly related to its length. Peripheral lines are wider and shorter than central lines and therefore offer much less resistance to flow. Central lines should be used only if peripheral lines cannot be started. Patients who are very unstable should have additional IV lines placed, ideally in the upper and lower extremities.

Fluid and Blood Administration

Initial fluid resuscitation consists of 2 liters of isotonic crystalloid fluid (lactated Ringer's or normal saline solution) given as a bolus over 15 to 60 minutes, depending on the severity of the situation. Use 2 liters for initial resuscitation because that amount should adequately resuscitate class I hemorrhagic shock (see Chapter 24, section on Hypovolemic and Hemorrhagic Shock). If hemodynamic instability develops or continues, severe hemorrhage is suspected, and additional fluid will be required.

Blood may be used for resuscitation in cases of class III or IV hemorrhagic shock. If blood is required immediately, type O-negative uncrossmatched blood is transfused (and is therefore available in the emergency rooms of all trauma centers). If it is possible to postpone transfusion, type-specific uncrossmatched or crossmatched blood can be available in 20 to 30 minutes.

ECG Monitoring

All patients are hooked up to ECG monitors to continuously assess heart rate as an index of the adequacy of resuscitation. An ECG may also detect arrhythmias, which may occur after myocardial contusion.

Nasogastric Tube Insertion

A nasogastric tube is inserted primarily to achieve gastric decompression and prevent aspiration. The detection of intragastric blood may also be noteworthy. Gastric decompression is also necessary if a peritoneal lavage is to be performed (see Chapter 21, section on

Diagnostic Peritoneal Lavage). In the patient with obvious or suspected maxillofacial trauma, the tube should be passed through the patient's mouth as an orogastric tube. *This prevents the possibility of passing the tube through an injured cribriform plate and into the brain!*

Foley Catheter Insertion

A Foley catheter is placed in all patients to decompress the bladder and follow hourly urine output as an index of adequacy of resuscitation. Before insertion of a Foley catheter in a male, the possibility of a urethral injury *must* be ruled out. (Urethral injuries in female trauma patients are rare because of the shorter urethra and absent prostate.) Ruling out urethral injury requires a rectal exam and visual inspection of the urethral meatus, scrotum, and perineum.

The presence of a high-riding, boggy, or nonpalpable prostate on digital rectal exam, blood at the urethral meatus, scrotal swelling or hematoma, or a perineal (often butterfly-shaped) hematoma all are signs consistent with urethral injury. In these cases, urologic consultation should be obtained to evaluate the lower genitourinary tract. This includes performing a retrograde urethrogram to find or rule out a urethral injury. If no injury is found, a Foley catheter can then be placed.

Additional workup for meatal blood includes a cystogram and intravenous pyelogram. If a urethral injury is present, options for bladder drainage include a percutaneous or surgically placed suprapubic catheter.

Lab Evaluation

A full panel of blood work is sent off during the initial evaluation, with the blood usually being collected through the initially placed IV. This includes a complete blood count, electrolyte panel, coagulation studies (PT and PTT), liver function studies, amylase and lipase, type and screen or cross match (for up to 6 units) as clinically indicated, ethanol level, and pregnancy test (β-human chorionic gonadotropin [HCG]) for women. A urine sample (usually obtained immediately after the

Foley catheter is placed) is tested for blood with a dip-stick and sent for full urinalysis and drug/toxicology screen.

SECONDARY SURVEY

During the secondary survey, a complete head-to-toe physical exam is performed, with special attention to traumatic injuries. Specifics of this exam, by system, include the following:

Head. The skull is palpated for depressed skull fractures. The eyes are examined for pupillary size and re-activity, taking note of asymmetry or nonreactivity. Subconjunctival hemorrhage and periorbital edema should signal the possibility of ocular injury or corneal abrasions. Otoscopic exam is essential to rule out hemotympanum. Nasal fractures can be palpated. The face and jaw are palpated firmly to rule out fractures.

Neck. Although most patients still have a cervical collar on at this time, the front part of it should be removed to perform the exam after the patient is advised not to move his or her neck. Palpate neck for crepitance, a sign of tracheal, esophageal, or lung (pneumothorax) injury. Presence of a midline trachea and carotid pulses is verified. The presence of jugular venous distention is noted. The posterior cervical spine is palpated to detect tenderness that may signify a spinal injury.

Chest. The chest is observed for symmetrical excursions with ventilation. The lungs are auscultated for normal bilateral breath sounds. Decreased breath sounds may be a sign of pneumothorax, hemothorax, or pulmonary contusion. The chest wall is palpated for crepitance, a sign of a likely pneumothorax. The heart is auscultated to ensure clear heart sounds. The ribs and clavicles are palpated to detect fractures.

Abdomen. The abdomen is observed for previous scars, distention, and ecchymoses. Thorough palpation is intended to detect tenderness, which may be a sign of intra-abdominal injury.

Rectum. A digital rectal exam is mandatory before Foley catheter placement in a male. Rectal sphincter tone is assessed, which may be decreased or absent in spinal cord injuries. The position and consistency of the prostate are assessed. The presence of gross blood may indicate a colon or rectal injury.

Extremities. The arms and legs are observed for gross deformities, swelling, ecchymoses, and abrasions. Long bones are palpated for fractures. When fractures or penetrating trauma involves an extremity, distal pulses and motor and sensory function must be documented. The pelvis is firmly rocked or pushed to assess its stability.

Neurologic screen. A full Glasgow Coma Scale (see Chapter 23, section on Closed Head Injuries) is recorded (although this is usually done earlier in the evaluation). At a minimum, the patient is asked to move all four extremities and exhibit normal sensation throughout. If a spinal cord injury is suspected, a sensory spinal level is determined. The patient is log-rolled onto one side, and the entire spine is palpated for tenderness.

Screening x-rays. PEARL: Three x-rays are mandatory in all trauma patients: lateral cervical spine, chest, and pelvis.

- The lateral C-spine film is done to rule out cervical spine injury. All seven cervical vertebrae must be seen, as well as the top of the body of T1, to begin clearing the C spine.
- The chest x-ray obtained at this time is a supine anteroposterior film. It is meant to detect subclinical pneumothorax or hemothorax, assess the mediastinal width, and check position of an endotracheal and nasogastric tube, if present.
- The pelvic x-ray is done to rule out pelvic fractures. These fractures mandate changing the location where a diagnostic peritoneal lavage is performed (see Chapter 21, section on Diagnostic Peritoneal Lavage).

SPECIAL SITUATIONS

Pediatric Trauma

Several caveats in the assessment and management of pediatric trauma are noteworthy:

- Normal vital signs are age-dependent with increased pulse and decreased blood pressure in younger children.

- Fluid resuscitation begins with a 20 mL/kg bolus of isotonic crystalloid fluid, which may be repeated up to three times as necessary.
- The evaluation of blunt abdominal trauma is almost exclusively done by CT scan, and nonoperative, expectant management of bleeding spleen and liver injuries is predominant.
- Bony fractures and their management are influenced by injury to the growth plates.

Trauma in Pregnancy

The most important determinant of fetal outcome is adequate and appropriate resuscitation and management of the traumatized pregnant patient. An appreciation of the altered vital signs and blood volume during pregnancy is important. Unless spinal injury is suspected, the pregnant patient should be evaluated while lying on her left side to avoid compression of the vena cava by the gravid uterus and resulting poor venous return to the heart. Fetal monitoring should be instituted early to detect fetal distress.

21
CHAPTER

Abdominal Trauma

GENERAL CONSIDERATIONS

The single most important determination in the management of abdominal trauma is not what the specific injury is but rather that an injury is or may be present and that operative intervention is required. Several basic facts are fundamental to making this determination:

1. The physical examination is often unreliable because many patients with significant injuries are asymptomatic. The frequent presence of altered mental status (as seen with closed head injury or alcohol use) precludes a meaningful examination. Therefore, diagnostic modalities such as computed tomography (CT) scan, diagnostic peritoneal lavage (DPL), ultrasound, and serial exam and observation are needed to supplement the evaluation.

2. The pathophysiology of blunt injury differs from that of penetrating injury.

   • In penetrating injuries, a further distinction must be made between stab wounds (low-energy) and gunshot wounds (GSWs) (high-energy with blast effect). For GSWs to the abdomen, the chance of serious hollow viscus (bowel) or other injury is high. Exploratory laparotomy is required for injuries that penetrate into the peritoneal cavity. For stab wounds, the incidence of injury is lower than for GSWs, and in certain cases there is a place for observation, DPL, or even diagnostic laparoscopy. **PEARL: Because of the high incidence of organ injury after GSWs to the abdomen, exploratory laparotomy is required.**

- For blunt trauma, the incidence of injury is low. The most commonly injured organs are the spleen and liver, where bleeding is usually the result. Therefore, the evaluation of blunt abdominal trauma is centered on determining the presence of intra-abdominal blood and whether there is enough bleeding to require exploratory laparotomy and possible repair of the source (Table 21–1).

3. The use of adjunctive diagnostic tests in the evaluation of abdominal trauma is primarily (and almost exclusively) designed for the patient with hemodynamic stability and either negative, equivocal, or unreliable physical examination. If the patient is hemodynamically unstable or has a physical exam that is highly suggestive of injury (peritoneal signs, moderate to severe diffuse tenderness, distention with dullness to percussion suggestive of a large hemoperitoneum), emergency exploratory laparotomy is indicated and further diagnostic testing is unwarranted.

BLUNT ABDOMINAL TRAUMA

The most common causes of blunt abdominal trauma are motor vehicle accidents, assaults, and falls.

Table 21–1. DIAGNOSTIC MODALITIES FOR EVALUATION OF BLUNT ABDOMINAL TRAUMA

CT scan
Diagnostic peritoneal lavage (DPL)
Ultrasound
Observation, serial exams, and lab tests

PEARL: The most commonly injured organs following blunt abdominal trauma are the spleen and liver. Most of these injuries can be managed nonoperatively. For many patients, one or more diagnostic procedures are required to rule in or out a significant intra-abdominal injury that might require laparotomy.

CT Scan

PEARL: The most widely used diagnostic test for blunt abdominal trauma is the CT scan. This is true because it is noninvasive, specific (pinpoints what organ is injured and to what degree), and fairly rapidly obtainable in most centers.

CT's disadvantages include high cost (when compared with DPL) and poor sensitivity and specificity for bowel injuries and perforations.

During CT scanning, oral contrast (usually given via the nasogastric tube) is used to outline the stomach and bowel. Intra-abdominal blood is seen as fluid in the pelvis or around the liver or spleen.

Grading systems have been developed for spleen and liver injuries. Such injuries range from minor subcapsular hematomas to major lacerations that involve devitalized tissue and hilar injury. These grading systems provide guidance in determining the need for operative intervention in the hemodynamically stable patient.

Diagnostic Peritoneal Lavage

DPL is a minor surgical procedure performed primarily because of its sensitivity in determining the presence of intra-abdominal blood in patients suspected of sustaining intra-abdominal injury from blunt trauma. Following is a description of the DPL procedure:

- A nasogastric or orogastric tube and Foley catheter must be in place to decompress the stomach and bladder, respectively.
- The technique involves inserting a small catheter into the peritoneal cavity, either via a small infra-umbilical midline incision or percutaneously, and

aspirating to detect blood. An initial aspirate of 5 to 10 mL of blood is considered positive. Aspiration of any enteric contents is also positive.
- If no blood (or less than 5 mL of blood) is aspirated, 1 L of normal saline or lactated Ringer's solution is infused through the catheter, and the fluid is then siphoned off to detect whether it became bloody by mixing with intraperitoneal blood.
- Samples of the lavaged fluid are sent for laboratory evaluation. Table 21–2 lists criteria for positive findings.

Table 21–2. CRITERIA FOR A POSITIVE DIAGNOSTIC PERITONEAL LAVAGE

>100,000 RBCs/mm^3
>500 WBCs/mm^3
Presence of bacteria, food, or fecal matter on Gram's stain
Elevated amylase, lipase, bilirubin

Most patients with an aspirate of gross blood go to surgery. Patients with a lavage positive by RBC count may have minor splenic and liver injuries that stopped bleeding on their own. Thus, a stable patient may undergo CT scanning and, if appropriate, may be managed nonoperatively.

PEARL: DPL should not be performed in the presence of a previous midline incision because of underlying bowel loop adhesions. In the presence of a pelvic fracture, a supraumbilical approach is recommended to avoid properitoneal blood that can dissect up the anterior abdominal wall to the level of the umbilicus.

A major disadvantage of DPL is its inability to detect injury to retroperitoneal organs (pancreas, duodenum) and its less than optimal sensitivity for injuries to bowel, diaphragm, and bladder.

Ultrasound

Ultrasound is becoming popular in the workup of blunt abdominal trauma, and its use will likely grow in the future. With ultrasound, intra-abdominal blood can be detected, and the nature of spleen and liver injuries can be defined. **PEARL: The major advantage of ultrasound is that it can be performed quickly and portably in the emergency room.** As experience with its use grows, ultrasound may replace CT scanning in many patients.

Observation, Serial Exams, and Lab Tests

In patients who have negative physical findings and where the index of suspicion for intra-abdominal injury is low, overnight observation with serial abdominal exams and follow-up labs is often appropriate. (This presumes that the physical examination is reliable in that the patient is neither obtunded nor intoxicated and does not require general anesthesia for management of other injuries.)

Spleen

In the past, splenectomy was commonly performed for splenic injuries, but it is uncommon now except for the most severe injuries. In fact, most splenic injuries are now managed nonoperatively and expectantly. In patients who fail nonoperative management (e.g., they become hemodynamically unstable or require more than 2 units of transfused blood) or who require initial operative intervention because of high-grade injuries or hemodynamic instability, repair of the spleen (splenorrhaphy) is indicated.

Mainstays of splenic repair include special suturing techniques and use of a wrapping mesh. A growing appreciation of the immunological importance of the spleen has fueled the trend of splenorrhaphy over splenectomy. If splenectomy is performed, patients must be immunized against *Pneumococcus* and *Hemophilus* with available vaccines to prevent postsplenectomy sepsis.

Liver and Other Organs

Most low-grade liver injuries can also be managed expectantly. High-grade injuries often require operative intervention using various methods to control bleeding, special suturing techniques, temporary packing, or, rarely, segmental resection.

Other less common blunt abdominal injuries include those to the diaphragm (usually tears on the left side that require suture repair), duodenum (ranging from hematomas that can be managed expectantly to perforations that require operative repair), and pancreas (from contusions, which can be managed expectantly, to transection, which requires operative repair). Patients with renal contusions usually present with microscopic hematuria and can be managed expectantly. (The presence of hematuria does require urological work-up with CT, intravenous pyelography, cystography, or urethrography to rule out other injuries.)

PENETRATING ABDOMINAL TRAUMA

PEARL: The most commonly injured organ following penetrating abdominal trauma is small bowel. Exploratory laparotomy is mandatory after GSWs, regardless of the patient's hemodynamic status. It is used selectively following stab wounds.

The incidence of significant injury after penetrating abdominal trauma is high, particularly after GSWs (about 95%). At times, it may be difficult to determine whether a bullet entered or crossed the peritoneal cavity, especially for wounds of the flank, pelvis, or chest. In these cases, adjunctive tests such as DPL, CT, diagnostic laparoscopy, or observation with serial exams may be warranted.

Stab wounds to the abdomen also carry a fairly high incidence of intra-abdominal injury, although not as high as GSWs. Therefore, in the presence of hemodynamic instability or obvious signs of injury (e.g., peritoneal signs, omental or bowel evisceration), laparotomy is indicated. Otherwise, adjunctive measures such as wound tract exploration (to determine whether peritoneal penetration occurred), DPL, diagnostic laparoscopy, or observation with serial exams may be used in lieu of exploratory laparotomy.

Because the most commonly injured organ after penetrating abdominal trauma is the small bowel, which does not bleed very much, the RBC criterium for DPL in these situations is modified. To improve its sensitivity in detecting injury, the RBC criterium is lowered to 10,000 to 20,000/mm³.

Management

After penetrating injury, most small-bowel injuries consist of small holes that can be repaired by primary suture closure. More extensive injuries may require resection with anastomosis. The following are treatment principles for various injuries sustained from penetrating trauma:

- Injuries to the large bowel can usually be managed by simple closure. Injuries involving the left colon and rectum often require creation of a colostomy to divert the fecal stream.
- Gastric injuries can be managed by suture closure.
- Vascular injuries within the abdomen require careful identification and isolation, followed by ligation, suture repair, or bypass as needed.
- Injuries to the diaphragm, which can occur after penetrating trauma to the chest or abdomen, require primary closure.
- Genitourinary injuries involving the ureters and bladder can be repaired primarily and may also require placement of a stent or suprapubic tube.

It is extremely important that during laparotomy for penetrating injuries a thorough and systematic exploration be done to avoid missing injuries that may be subtle.

22
CHAPTER

Thoracic Trauma

Only 10 to 15% of thoracic injuries require surgical intervention. **PEARL: Eighty-five to 90% of thoracic injuries can be managed by chest tube placement alone.** Major life-threatening thoracic injuries including tension pneumothorax, open pneumothorax, flail chest, and cardiac tamponade (discussed in Chapter 20, section on Primary Survey) must be recognized and treated during the primary survey. The thoracic injuries discussed in the following sections are usually identified during the secondary survey and are treated during this time or during the definitive care phase.

MASSIVE HEMOTHORAX

Massive hemothorax usually results from penetrating thoracic trauma and is defined by 1500 mL or more of blood in a thoracic cavity.

Diagnostic findings for massive hemothorax include:

- Hypoxia
- Hemodynamic instability (heart rate >100; systolic blood pressure <90)
- Absence of breath sounds or dullness to percussion on one side of the chest
- Possible distention of neck veins (due to mechanical effects on the mediastinum) or flatness of neck veins (due to hypovolemia)

Chest x-ray should not be necessary to make the diagnosis of massive hemothorax. Management requires placement of a large-bore (38 French) chest tube.

PEARL: Indications for exploratory thoracotomy: initial blood loss of ≥1500 mL or continued blood loss through the chest tube at a rate of ≥200 mL or more per hour.

Smaller hemothoraces are usually diagnosed after the initial chest x-ray is obtained. Tube thoracostomy is required in all such cases to evacuate the blood and prevent subsequent development of a fibrothorax and its resulting constrictive component.

PULMONARY CONTUSION

Pulmonary contusion occurs when a segment of lung is "bruised," usually by blunt chest wall trauma and occasionally by the direct blast effect of a gunshot wound (GSW). In the setting of blunt chest trauma, overlying rib fractures are usually present. The resulting intra-alveolar and interstitial hemorrhage and fluid exudation cause a ventilation-perfusion mismatch and result in varying degrees of hypoxia.

The chest x-ray usually demonstrates a localized infiltrate, but this radiographic picture may take up to 24 hours to develop.

Depending on the severity, management of pulmonary contusion may range from observation with oxygen supplementation to the need for endotracheal intubation and positive pressure mechanical ventilation. In the more severe cases, the clinical picture is similar to that of the patient with adult respiratory distress syndrome (ARDS).

MYOCARDIAL CONTUSION

Myocardial contusion results from blunt thoracic trauma that bruises the heart. This usually occurs in a motor vehicle accident (MVA) in which an unrestrained driver is thrown into the steering wheel, resulting in rapid compression of the heart between the sternum and the thoracic spine.

Presenting signs vary from none, to arrhythmias, to cardiogenic shock. **PEARL: Diagnosis of myocardial contusion is aided by ECG (arrhythmias, acute injury pattern), serial cardiac enzymes (elevated CK-MB fraction and index, elevated troponin), and echocardiography (ventricular wall hypokinesis).**

Depending on the severity, management of myocardial contusion varies from 24-hour observation with cardiac monitoring to hemodynamic monitoring and support similar to that for a patient with an acute myocardial infarction. **PEARL: Most documented myocardial contusions resolve spontaneously without sequelae.**

TRAUMATIC AORTIC RUPTURE

Traumatic aortic rupture or tear results from decelerating injuries such as MVAs and falls. The pathophysiology most commonly involves a tear of the descending thoracic aorta at the level of the ligamentum arteriosum, a spot where tethering on the aorta makes it more vulnerable to shear. Traumatic aortic rupture is the most common cause of sudden death after an MVA. **PEARL: Of patients with traumatic aortic rupture, 90% die at the scene because of exsanguinating hemorrhage.**

Of the 10% of patients with traumatic aortic rupture who arrive at the hospital alive—usually with partial or contained tears—mortality is high if the condition is not recognized and treated. A high index of suspicion must be maintained in patients who have sustained significant decelerating injuries and have one or more radiographic signs on chest x-ray, as listed in Table 22–1.

PEARL: The most consistent and commonly encountered radiographic finding in a patient with traumatic aortic rupture is a widened mediastinum. The initial chest x-ray is a supine anteroposterior film, which tends to magnify the mediastinum. If a widened mediastinum is the only sign, an upright posteroanterior film should be obtained after the cervical spine is cleared (if clinically appropriate) so that the width of the mediastinum can be confirmed.

To confirm or exclude the diagnosis of traumatic aortic rupture, a thoracic aortogram is required (and is considered the gold standard). If the proper level of suspicion is maintained, the rate of positive findings for

Table 22–1. CHEST X-RAY FINDINGS ASSOCIATED WITH TRAUMATIC AORTIC RUPTURE

Widened mediastinum: >8 cm on upright PA film
Fractures of the first and second ribs
Obliteration of the aortic knob
Deviation of the trachea to the right
Presence of a pleural cap (blood beneath the parietal pleura at the lung apex)
Elevation and rightward shift of the right mainstem bronchus
Depression of the left mainstem bronchus
Obliteration of the aortopulmonary window
Deviation of the esophagus (nasogastric tube) to the right

traumatic aortic rupture on aortograms should be about 10% (90% of aortograms are negative).

For a patient undergoing CT scans to evaluate the head or abdomen, a chest CT with IV contrast is an appropriate alternative in selected low-risk cases. However, if the CT scan is positive or suspicious, a follow-up aortogram is required.

Definitive management of traumatic aortic rupture requires thoracotomy with either primary repair or resection and repair with a vascular graft.

OTHER INJURIES

Traumatic Diaphragmatic Hernia

Traumatic diaphragmatic hernias due to blunt trauma are usually large and typically on the left side. (The right diaphragm is protected by the liver.) These injuries should be suspected in patients with chest radiographic abnormalities of the left hemidiaphragm (elevated) or left chest (e.g., with loculated pneumohemothorax, gastric or colonic air pattern above the diaphragm, or nasogastric tube curled in chest). When such a hernia is due to penetrating injuries, the injury is usually small and is suspected based on the projectile's trajectory or is found at the time of laparotomy.

Treatment of traumatic diaphragmatic hernia consists of surgical repair—almost always via a laparotomy because of the high incidence of associated intra-abdominal injuries.

Tracheobronchial Tree Injuries

Tracheobronchial injuries are usually the result of penetrating injury. The following are possible manifestations of these injures:

- Signs of airway compromise
- Hemoptysis
- Subcutaneous emphysema
- Pneumothorax
- Large air leak through a chest tube

Tracheal injuries are often associated with injury of other structures (e.g., esophagus, carotid artery, jugular vein). Fiber-optic bronchoscopy is helpful in the diagnosis. Treatment requires surgical repair.

Esophageal Trauma

Injuries to the esophagus are almost always caused by penetrating trauma. Esophageal trauma is suspected in patients with the following:

- Pneumothorax or hemothorax without associated rib fractures
- Particulate matter appearing in chest tube drainage
- Mediastinal air

Confirmation usually is made with x-ray (gastrograffin swallow) or esophagoscopy. Treatment of esophageal trauma requires surgical repair and wide drainage of the mediastinum and pleural space.

Simple Pneumothorax

Pneumothorax most frequently results from blunt trauma and laceration of the lung by rib fractures, less commonly from penetrating trauma. Most pneumothoraces do not progress to cause tension and are discovered either on chest radiography or physical exam (subcutaneous emphysema, chest wall crepitation, decreased breath sounds). **PEARL: Once traumatic pneumothorax is suspected or diagnosed—no matter how small—a chest tube should always be placed.**

Rib Fractures

Rib fractures are the most common thoracic injury and almost always result from blunt trauma. Diagnosis of rib fracture is usually made on physical exam with the following findings:

- Localized pain and tenderness
- Palpation of bony crepitation

Rib fracture is a clinical diagnosis, and rib x-rays are therefore superfluous. Chest x-ray is important to ascertain whether an associated pneumothorax or hemothorax is present.

When there are no associated thoracic injuries, management of rib fracture is directed toward pain control to prevent splinting, atelectasis, and progression to pneumonia. Adequate pain control allows for better pulmonary toilet, cough and deep breathing, and incentive spirometry. Measures for control of pain include the following:

- Oral or intramuscular analgesics
- IV patient-controlled analgesia (PCA: morphine or meperidine pump)
- Rib blocks with long-acting local anesthetics
- Pleural catheters
- Thoracic epidural catheters

EMERGENCY ROOM THORACOTOMY

The main indication for emergency room thoracotomy is in the patient with penetrating trauma to the chest who loses vital signs in the ER or shortly before arrival during transport. Although the indications and success of emergency room thoracotomy ("cracking a chest") are limited, the following comments on this topic are appropriate.

- After tension pneumothorax is ruled out (by thrusting 14-gauge needles into both chests), the left chest is opened with a thoracotomy incision along the fifth interspace and a rib spreader is placed.
- The goal of emergency thoracotomy is to identify and control one of several rapidly correctable life-threatening injuries, such as pericardial tamponade or hilar lung injury. In these cases, therapy includes opening the pericardial sac to relieve tamponade, holding pressure on a bleeding cardiac injury, or clamping a lung hilum to control bleeding.
- Other therapeutic maneuvers may include clamping the descending thoracic aorta (useful to control massive intra-abdominal bleeding that resulted in arrest) and beginning open cardiac massage.
- If a positive response results, the patient is immediately taken to the operating room for continued resuscitation and definitive care.

PEARL: Cardiac arrest and loss of vital signs due to blunt trauma carries an almost 100% fatality rate and only rarely is ER thoracotomy indicated.

23
CHAPTER

Trauma of the Head, Neck, and Extremities

The multidisciplinary trauma team is frequently faced with patients with multiple injuries. The problems discussed in this chapter include head and neck injuries, injuries to the extremities, and central nervous system injuries.

HEAD INJURIES

Closed Head Injuries

Closed head injuries consist of blunt trauma to the head and are usually sustained during motor vehicle accidents (MVAs). **PEARL: Loss of consciousness, altered mental status, and decreased Glasgow Coma Scale (GCS) are common findings in closed head injury.**

The degree of neurological impairment is quantified by means of the GCS. The GCS assessment covers neurological responses in three areas: eye, verbal, and motor responses. The scale ranges from 3 (no responses) to 15 (normal). Severe closed head injuries are classified as 8 or lower.

Initial measures in closed head–injured patients are aimed at preventing and minimizing increases in intracranial pressure that result from brain edema within the cranium. These measures include the following:

- Hyperventilation (requiring intubation and mechanical ventilation) to lower the $PaCO_2$ to 25 to 30 mm Hg
- Avoiding fluid excesses
- Promoting a diuresis (if tolerable)

PEARL: The single most important diagnostic test in the management of closed head trauma is the CT scan. It allows for the identification of intracranial injuries that often require operative intervention (depressed skull fracture, epidural hematoma, subdural hematoma) versus those injuries that are managed expectantly (contusion, diffuse axonal injury, subarachnoid hemorrhage). Management may also require monitoring of intracranial pressure by means of a subarachnoid bolt or intraventricular catheter. Early neurosurgical consultation is advised.

Gunshot Wounds

Gunshot wounds to the head are associated with high morbidity and mortality. Through-and-through injuries and those involving the lower brain and brain stem are most ominous. Skull x-rays and CT scan are usually obtained to determine whether any surgical intervention is necessary.

Spinal Cord Injuries

Spinal cord injuries must be suspected in all patients suffering blunt trauma. **PEARL: Spinal immobilization, especially to the cervical spine, is maintained until injury can be ruled out.** Paralysis, sensory levels, and other neurological findings are sought.

Cervical spine films can be supplemented by films of the thoracic and lumbosacral spine as needed. CT is also indicated to define the exact nature of any injuries. **Spinal shock** or **neurogenic shock** refers to the clinical syndrome of hypotension due to peripheral vasodilatation, which results from cervical or high thoracic spinal cord injury. Patients also often have bradycardia. **PEARL: Cervical and other spinal cord injuries must be suspected in all blunt trauma patients. They are ruled out by x-rays and neurological examination.**

Treatment of the spinal cord–injured patient consists of leg elevation to promote venous return and fluid resuscitation. Atropine may be used to reverse bradycardia and phenylephrine to reverse vasodilatation, if needed. Early neurosurgical or orthopedic consultation is warranted to plan definitive management.

PENETRATING NECK TRAUMA

Penetrating trauma to the neck requires careful evaluation because of the high density of vital structures within a relatively small area. After it is determined that a wound has penetrated the platysma muscle layer, which either is obvious or requires careful exploration, the underlying injuries are the next concern. At times, a patient has obvious physical evidence of injury with an expanding or large hematoma, airway compromise, or crepitation. Most often, however, this is not the case, and injuries to vital structures must be sought and confirmed or ruled out.

The evaluation and management of penetrating neck injuries in the absence of obvious physical signs are determined by the specific location or zone of injury in the neck. The neck is divided into three zones (Fig. 23–1).

- **Zone I** is the region below a line drawn across the cricoid cartilage. This zone extends down to the suprasternal notch and the thoracic inlet.
- **Zone III** is the area above a horizontal line drawn from the angle of the mandible. This area extends up to the skull base.
- **Zone II** is the largest area and constitutes everything between zones I and III.

Because of the inherent difficulties in surgical exposure and proximal (in zone I) and distal (in zone III) control of vessels in zone I and zone III, injuries in these areas are evaluated by a combination of arteriography (to assess carotid and vertebral arteries), gastrograffin

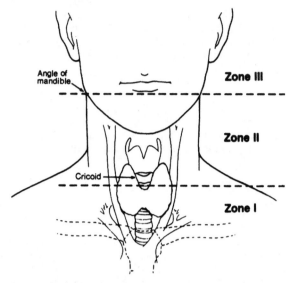

Figure 23–1. Zones of the neck (From Thal E.R. Injury to the neck. In Feliciano, DV, Moore, EE, Mattox, KL [eds]: Trauma, ed 3. Appleton & Lange, Stamford, Conn., 1996, p 330, with permission.)

and barium swallow (to evaluate the esophagus), and bronchoscopy (to evaluate the trachea). Identified injuries are then managed surgically.

Because of the easy surgical exposure and control abilities within zone II, these injuries are evaluated and managed by surgical neck exploration. There is a trend toward a more selective approach to zone II injuries in some centers.

PEARL: Penetrating trauma to the neck is usually managed with surgical neck exploration for zone II injuries and selective exploration after diagnostic workup for zone I and zone III injuries.

EXTREMITY TRAUMA

Injuries to the extremities are primarily orthopedic and vascular in nature. Fractures can occur from blunt trauma as well as from gunshot wounds. Usually, fractures from blunt trauma can be recognized on physical exam by an obvious deformity or localized pain. Definitive diagnosis is obtained by x-ray.

Management

Fractures

PEARL: Initial ER management of fractures includes splinting and assessment for associated vascular injury. Splinting limits both bleeding and pain. Assessment of distal pulses in all fractured extremities is essential because some fractures are associated with major arterial injuries.

Fractures with an associated break in the skin are classified as *open fractures* and are surgical emergencies. They require operative cleansing and bone stabilization once other life-threatening injuries are ruled out or managed. In general, the trend is toward early ORIF (operative reduction and internal fixation) of all major long bone fractures.

Vascular Injuries

Vascular injuries are usually the result of penetrating trauma. Some injuries are obvious on physical exam:

- Large or expanding hematoma
- Excessive bleeding through the wound
- Absent distal pulses
- A perfusion-compromised extremity

These injuries require immediate operative exploration. Injuries without obvious signs may be suspected based on proximity to major vessels, diminished pulses, or an abnormally low ankle-brachial index (ratio of systolic blood pressure in the dorsalis pedis to brachial artery as measured by Doppler). **PEARL: In the absence of obvious physical signs, suspected arterial injuries are evaluated by arteriography.** Operative repair of arterial injuries may consist of the following:

- Suture repair
- Resection and primary anastomosis or grafting with either autogenous vein or prosthetic grafts

24
CHAPTER

Shock

The diagnosis and management of shock remain major problems in the care of many surgical patients. Although patients in shock often receive the most intensive care, they have extremely high levels of morbidity and mortality. Proper management of shock includes the following:

- Rapid diagnosis
- Aggressive resuscitation
- Correction of the underlying cause

This chapter focuses on the diagnosis, classification and etiology, and management of shock, as well as its complications.

DEFINITION

Physicians and physiologists have struggled for over a century to develop a unifying definition of shock. Modern definitions tend to stress the patient as a whole, emphasize vital organ function, and focus on the lack of adequate blood flow, or perfusion, to vital organs and tissues. **PEARL: A shock state exists when there is inadequate tissue perfusion.** More broadly, a shock state exists when the circulation fails to meet the nutritional needs of the cells, and fails to remove metabolic wastes.

A diagnosis of shock is often simplistically considered in patients who have a low blood pressure, but this cannot be the sole diagnostic criterion. Patients with normal blood pressure can manifest many of the signs, symptoms, and sequelae of shock. In fact, when we refer to shock, we are really describing what happens to our patients after they suffer some type of catastrophic insult to their bodies.

CLINICAL MANIFESTATIONS

Many of the clinical manifestations of a patient with shock are unique to the specific cause of the shock. However, some general signs and symptoms are common to many, if not all, forms of shock, including the following:

- Hemodynamic instability: systolic blood pressure <90, heart rate >100, or both
- Altered mental status: lethargy, confusion
- Decreased urine output: less than 0.5 mL/kg/hr
- Skin: decreased capillary refill, cool, clammy skin

CLASSIFICATION

Although there are many different classifications of shock, a most useful classification categorizes shock according to the underlying system that is abnormal or dysfunctional (Table 24–1).

Cardiogenic Shock

In cardiogenic shock, the heart is unable to pump blood to meet the needs of the body. Hallmarks of this form of shock include the following:

Table 24–1. CLASSIFICATION OF SHOCK

Type of Shock	System Dysfunction
Cardiogenic	Heart (pump)
Hypovolemic/hemorrhagic	Fluid volume (tank)
Septic	Inflammation
Neurogenic	Arterial and venous tone

- Hypotension due to poor cardiac function (increased cardiac filling pressures, low cardiac output)
- Compensatory peripheral vasoconstriction
- Jugular venous distention (common)
- Elevated central venous pressure (CVP) and pulmonary artery wedge pressure if invasive hemodynamic monitoring (pulmonary artery catheter) is in place

Causes

The most common cause of cardiogenic shock is an acute myocardial infarction (MI). Although patients with cardiogenic shock are usually on the medical service, surgeons confront patients with known or silent myocardial ischemia who develop perioperative MIs during or after major surgery. In the arena of trauma, important causes of cardiogenic shock include pericardial tamponade and cardiac contusion. Some of the common causes of cardiogenic shock are listed in Table 24–2.

Treatment

In addition to general supportive measures, specific therapy for cardiogenic shock must be tailored to the underlying cause. For an MI, therapy includes:

- Nitrates to improve coronary blood flow
- Preload and afterload reduction to decrease cardiac work
- Inotropic support
- Insertion of an intra-aortic balloon pump (IABP) in refractory cases

Table 24–2. CAUSES OF CARDIOGENIC SHOCK

Myocardial infarction
Pericardial tamponade
Cardiac contusion
Arrhythmias
Pulmonary embolism
Cardiomyopathy
Chronic valvular disease
Postinfarction complications

In addition, pericardial tamponade in the setting of trauma is a surgical emergency and requires pericardiocentesis or subxiphoid pericardial window and open cardiac surgery.

Cardiac contusion is managed similarly to MI, but usually without nitrates.

Arrhythmias require accurate diagnosis and pharmacologic or electrical cardioversion.

Hypovolemic and Hemorrhagic Shock

In hypovolemic and hemorrhagic shock, the primary problem is insufficient volume in the circulation (i.e., the tank is not filled). The intravascular volume deficit can be due to loss of plasma volume or of blood. Common causes of hypovolemic shock include:

- Conditions that result in dehydration, such as vomiting (gastric outlet obstruction)
- Diarrhea (gastroenteritis)
- Third-space losses (paralytic ileus, bowel obstruction)
- Acute traumatic blood loss

When the body senses a state of hypovolemia, a number of compensatory responses are activated that help the patient cope with the hypovolemia and help us recognize the diagnosis and its severity. Table 24–3 lists these compensatory mechanisms and their sequelae.

When hypovolemic shock is due to hemorrhage, the severity of the shock is related to the percentage of total blood volume lost. This can be estimated by recognition of clinical parameters that are manifestations of of these compensatory mechanisms. Stratifying patients to a class of shock allows better tailoring of fluid and blood resuscitation (Table 24–4).

Treatment Principles

PEARL: The initial management of hypovolemic shock is prompt and aggressive fluid resuscitation.

**Table 24–3. COMPENSATORY
MECHANISMS IN HYPOVOLEMIC SHOCK
AND THEIR SEQUELAE**

Mechanism	Sequelae
Adrenergic discharge	Increases heart rate, peripheral vasoconstriction
Hyperventilation	Decreases CO_2 (controls acidosis)
Collapse	Redistributes blood from extremities
Release of vasoactive hormones (vasopressin)	Decreases urine output
Resorption of fluid from the interstitium	Restores intravascular volume
Shift of fluids from cells	Restores extracellular fluid
Renal conservation of water and electrolytes	Decreases urine output

- For hypovolemic shock without blood loss, fluid resuscitation with an isotonic crystalloid solution (either lactated Ringer's solution or normal saline) should begin with a 1- to 2-L bolus over no more than 60 minutes through two large-bore peripheral IV lines.
- Subsequent fluid resuscitation should be with the same isotonic crystalloid solution at a rate exceeding maintenance fluids, or 150 mL or more per hour (see Chapter 4).
- In the setting of acute blood loss, initial fluid resuscitation must also begin with a 2-L isotonic crystalloid bolus over about 15 to 30 minutes, depending on the severity of shock. **PEARL: Isotonic crystalloid fluid requirements in the resuscitation of hemorrhagic shock are estimated as three times the blood loss (3:1 rule).**
- Transfusion of blood (packed red blood cells) in the resuscitation phase is reserved for patients with class III or IV hemorrhagic shock and should not be used for lesser levels of shock. For this reason, uncrossmatched O-negative blood is kept in the ER of trauma hospitals, although type-specific or

Table 24–4. CLASSES OF HEMORRHAGIC SHOCK

	Class I	Class II	Class III	Class IV
Blood loss (mL)	<750	750–1500	1500–2000	>2000
Blood loss (% blood volume)	<15	15–30	30–40	>40
Pulse rate	<100	>100	>120	>140
Systolic BP	Normal	Normal	<90	<90
Capillary refill test	Normal	Positive	Positive	Positive
Respiratory rate	14–20	20–30	30–40	>35
Urine output (mL/hr)	>30	20–30	5–15	Negligible
Mental status	Slightly anxious	Mildly anxious	Anxious, confused	Confused, lethargic

Adapted from ACS Committee on Trauma, *Advanced Trauma Life Support® Student Manual,* 1993 Edition. Chicago, American College of Surgeons, 1993:86.

crossmatched blood can usually be ready in 20 to 30 minutes.

- Ongoing bleeding due to a traumatic injury requires operative intervention for definitive control.

Septic Shock

Septic shock results from sepsis or infection. The infectious agents that most commonly cause septic shock are gram-negative bacilli. Their endotoxins or lipopolysaccharides (LPS) have been identified as a common etiologic agent. However, these syndromes can also result from infection with gram-positive organisms, fungi, and viruses.

PEARL: Septic shock is characterized by hypotension and a low systemic vascular resistance (due to vasodilatation and shunting), along with an increased cardiac output (hyperdynamic state) up to two to three times normal.

Together, this results in a state of inadequate tissue perfusion.

The diagnosis of septic shock must be suspected in any patient with shock plus signs and symptoms of infection—fever, leukocytosis, bacteremia. In the surgical setting, common causes of septic shock include peritonitis (perforated peptic ulcer, perforated diverticulitis, perforated appendicitis) and nosocomial pneumonias. The hyperdynamic state may be diagnosed by inserting a pulmonary artery catheter, which allows measurement of cardiac output and systemic vascular resistance.

Treatment Principles

PEARL: Aggressive and rapid volume resuscitation must always precede surgical intervention for septic shock.

- The management of septic shock requires initial resuscitation of the patient with isotonic crystalloid solutions such as lactated Ringer's solution or normal saline.
- Aggressive antibiotics are initiated promptly and are tailored toward the suspected infection.
- When the underlying septic process requires surgical intervention (e.g., in the case of secondary peritonitis, most cases of tertiary peritonitis), the patient must be rapidly prepared for surgery (e.g., exploratory laparotomy with closure of a perforation, resection of diseased or nonviable bowel and irrigation of the peritoneal cavity, drainage of intra-abdominal abscess). It is important not to rush a patient to the operating room before adequate resuscitation has been completed. This resuscitation must proceed quickly so as not to delay the needed surgery.

Neurogenic Shock

Neurogenic (or spinal) shock is caused by the sudden loss of autonomic innervation of the vasculature, which results in vasodilatation of the entire vascular bed. **PEARL: Neurogenic shock is characterized by hypotension** due to peripheral vasodilatation that results from denervation of the vasculature.

Causes

Many clinical situations can cause neurogenic shock. Examples are traumatic cervical spinal cord injury, high spinal anesthesia, and vasovagal discharge.

Traumatic Spinal Cord Injuries

Spinal cord injuries usually result from automobile, bicycle, or (shallow water) diving accidents. Patients with traumatic spinal cord injuries typically present with a definite spinal motor and sensory deficit level, which localizes the injury or transection level to the cervical cord. Typical signs and symptoms of shock from spinal cord injury include the following:

- Flaccid paralysis
- Absence of normal rectal sphincter tone
- Absence of reflexes
- Hypotension (usually) with variable tachycardia
- Warm skin, rather than cold and clammy, because of the lack of compensatory peripheral vasoconstriction (secondary to denervation)
- Normal mental status (usually), unlike in other forms of shock
- Low systemic vascular resistance (if measured with a pulmonary artery catheter)

High Spinal Anesthesia

Neurogenic shock can be associated with spinal anesthesia. Hypotension can result from the peripheral vasodilatation caused by the anesthetic effect of the spinal medication. Usually, any hypotension associated with spinal anesthesia is transient and minimal because its effects are limited to the lower body. However, on rare occasions if a spinal anesthetic is administered at too high a level (e.g., high thoracic) or the medication migrates up the spinal cord (e.g., to the cervical level), a neurogenic shock state can result.

Vasovagal Discharge

Intense vasovagal discharge can also cause enough vasodilatation and bradycardia to result in a neurogenic shock–like state. This may occur when a person is overcome with grief upon learning of the death of a loved one. The vasovagal discharge initiated from the emotional distress causes peripheral vasodilatation to the point that blood pools in the extremities, and the person becomes hypotensive and may even faint.

Massive acute gastric dilatation can also trigger enough vasovagal discharge to lead to hypotension. (This form of shock is best managed by emergent insertion of a nasogastric tube to achieve gastric decompression).

Treatment

The treatment of neurogenic shock is aggressive isotonic crystalloid resuscitation. This serves to expand the intravascular volume to a size appropriate to the dilated vascular bed and thus restore adequate perfusion. Only when shock is persistent despite adequate resuscitation do we resort to vasopressors (i.e., phenylephrine [Neosynephrine]) to counteract the vasodilatation.

GENERAL MANAGEMENT

The management of shock begins with its recognition. Once diagnosed, the most important **initial management** involves the ABCs:

- Ensuring that the patient has an adequate, protected airway
- Ensuring that the patient is breathing or being ventilated
- Adequate assessment (BP, HR) and initial support (IV fluids) of the circulation

PEARL: The management of shock begins with the ABCs of life support. Shock management is then tailored toward its specific etiology, as shown in Table 24–5.

Table 24–5. GENERAL TREATMENT OF SHOCK STATES

Type of Shock	Treatment
Cardiogenic	
Myocardial infarction	Coronary vasodilators
	Diuresis (preload and afterload reduction)
Cardiac tamponade	Pericardiocentesis, pericardial window
	Surgery to correct underlying cardiac injury
Hypovolemic	Isotonic crystalloid resuscitation
Hemorrhagic	Isotonic crystalloid resuscitation
	Blood if loss ≥30% total blood volume
Septic	Isotonic crystalloid resuscitation
	Surgery to drain pus or resolve perforation
	Antibiotics
Neurogenic	Isotonic crystalloid resuscitation

All patients with shock should be cared for in an intensive care unit. This facilitates the increased physiologic monitoring that these patients often require (see Chapter 28). **Increased monitoring** in patients with shock often includes the following:

- Bladder (Foley) catheterization—to allow for hourly urine outputs as an important indicator of end-organ (kidney) perfusion.
- Pulse oximetry—to continually monitor arterial oxygen saturation. Remember that these cutaneous sensing devices are often inaccurate in hypoperfused and cold patients.
- Arterial line (A-line)—to allow for real-time, ongoing blood pressure measurement, particularly to assess response to inotropic or vasopressor therapy; also to allow for necessary blood drawing for determination of labs and arterial blood gases.
- Central venous pressure (CVP) monitoring—often placed to aid fluid resuscitation and monitor CVP.

CONTROVERSY: CVP measurements are subject to many variables in interpretation and should often not be solely relied on.

- Pulmonary artery (Swan-Ganz) catheterization—to assess the adequacy of whole body perfusion and calculate intrapulmonary shunt fractions in severely ill patients who require measurement of right heart filling pressures, pulmonary capillary wedge pressure as a reflection of left-sided heart pressures, cardiac output, systemic vascular resistance, and sampling of mixed venous blood (from the pulmonary artery).

Many patients with shock require pharmacologic support of the circulation in addition to fluid resuscitation. This may take the form of inotropes, vasopressors, or vasodilators (Table 24–6).

Other **supportive** therapeutic modalities are occasionally necessary for patients in shock:

Table 24–6. COMMON CARDIOVASCULAR AGENTS

Agent	Dose Range (μg/kg/min)	Other Major Effects
Inotropes		
Dopamine	2–15	Renal/mesenteric vasodilation at low doses
Dobutamine	2–15	Vasodilation
Amrinone	5–15	Vasodilation
Vasopressors		
Norepinephrine	0.05–0.2	Inotrope
Epinephrine	0.03–0.2	Inotrope/chronotrope at low doses
Phenylephrine	0.6–2	Pure alpha vasoconstrictor
Vasodilators		
Nitroglycerin	0.2–2	Coronary vasodilation
Nitroprusside	1–5	Pure vasodilator

- Ventilatory support
- Nutritional support (enteral or parenteral nutrition)
- Stress gastritis prophylaxis
- Hemodialysis and hemofiltration
- Immunotherapy (cytokine, anticytokine or antiendotoxin therapies)—awaiting clinical confirmation of efficacy

COMPLICATIONS

With the great advances in intensive care over the past decade, we are often successful in reversing the hemodynamic effects of shock. In fact, a patient rarely dies of the initial shock state. However, some patients do die from end-organ manifestations of shock, which may develop despite reversal of the hemodynamic picture. These manifestations collectively are termed multisystem organ failure (MSOF) or multiple organ failure syndrome. These MSOF complications include:

- Acute renal failure
- Adult respiratory distress syndrome (ARDS)
- Hepatic failure
- Coagulopathy
- Stress gastritis
- Gut dysfunction
- Immune dysfunction

PEARL: Infections are the leading cause of death after management of shock.

25
CHAPTER

Burns

Burn injury represents a major traumatic insult to the body's largest organ—the skin. It results in a tremendous inflammatory response as well as compromise of the skin's vital function in fluid homeostasis. Care of burn patients presents some unique challenges related to these derangements.

Burn care can be divided into three stages:

1. The acute injury resuscitation phase
2. The burn wound care phase
3. The rehabilitation phase

RESUSCITATION

Basic Principles

The following are guidelines for resuscitation of a patient with burns:

1. Stop the burning process by extinguishing the source and removing all burned clothing. Apply moist clean towels if the wound is small or wrap the patient in a dry drape. No ointments are used at this time.
2. Protect the airway. Many patients are able to talk during the initial postinjury period. If the burn is full thickness, they may not have significant pain. Obtain a quick history of medications, allergies, and illnesses and explain what you're going to do. Consider

early intubation if inhalation injury is suspected. The airway soon becomes edematous both from direct thermal injury and fluid resuscitation. Administer oxygen to the patient.

3. Establish secure IV access. At least two large-bore peripheral IVs are needed. The IV may be placed through the burn wound if necessary. Place a nasogastric tube and a Foley catheter in patients with burns over more than 20% of their total body surface area. Urine output is one guide to adequate fluid resuscitation.

4. Rule out other injuries, especially if there is associated trauma.

Attention to the basic principles of trauma resuscitation and the timely application of emergency burn treatment will reduce morbidity and mortality from burn injury.

Burn complications include renal failure, sepsis, and airway compromise. They are aggravated by delayed recognition of the problem and delayed or inadequate fluid resuscitation. **PEARL: Delay in appropriate treatment is the most common cause of complications in severe burn injuries.**

Assessment and Stabilization

Airway and breathing are the initial concerns with the burn patient. The supraglottic airway is extremely susceptible to obstruction from heat exposure. Inhalation of carbon products and toxic fumes leads to a chemical tracheobronchitis and edema.

Indicators of inhalation injury include:

- Facial burns
- Singed eyebrows and nasal passages
- Carbon deposits or acute inflammation in the oropharynx
- History of mental impairment
- History of explosion or fire in a confined space.

PEARL: When in doubt, intubate!

Carbon monoxide injury should always be assumed when fire occurs in a closed space. Carbon monoxide has 240 times as great an affinity for hemoglobin as does oxygen. It therefore displaces oxygen from the hemoglobin molecule.

Baseline carboxyhemoglobin levels should be obtained, and patients should be started on 100% oxygen. The half-life of carbon monoxide is 250 minutes on room air and 40 minutes on 100% oxygen. Arterial PO_2 measurements are not a reliable indicator of carbon monoxide poisoning. A carbon monoxide partial pressure of only 1 mm Hg results in a carboxyhemoglobin level of greater than 40%. This is associated with changes in mental status.

Burn Surface Area

The burn surface area is used to guide initial therapy. A useful and practical guide to determine the extent of injury is the "rule of nines" (Fig. 25–1). In an adult, the total body surface area can be divided into anatomic regions that represent 9% or multiples of 9% as follows:

Each upper limb	9%
Each lower limb	18%
Anterior trunk	18%
Posterior trunk	18%
Head and neck	9%
Perineum and genitalia	1%

PEARL: The rule of nines does not apply to infants and young children. The total body surface represented by an infant's head is twice that represented by an adult's head. For children with smaller burns, the burn size can be estimated by using the patient's palm (not including fingers) to represent 1% of body surface.

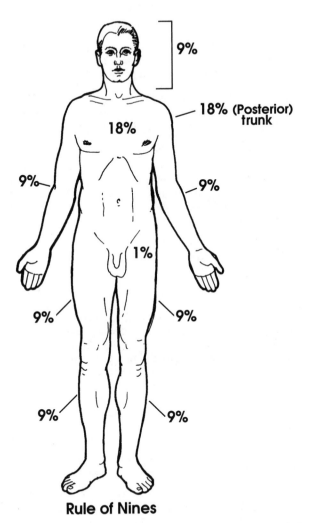

9%

18% (Posterior) trunk

18%

9%

9%

1%

9%

9%

9%

9%

Rule of Nines

Figure 25–1. The rule of nines allows rapid estimation of body surface area covered by burns. Note that each leg includes 9% for the lower and 9% for the upper leg.

Depth of Burn

The depth of the burn is an important factor in evaluating its severity. For example:

- First-degree burns (e.g., sunburn) are characterized by erythema, pain, and lack of blisters. Only the epidermis is involved.
- Second-degree or partial-thickness burns have a matted appearance, have blister formation, usually appear wet, and are exquisitely painful. The epidermis and varying levels of dermis are involved.
- Third-degree or full-thickness burns appear dark and leathery or translucent and waxy white. These burns are often dry and pain-free because the pain receptors are damaged. All skin layers including skin appendages, blood vessels, and nerve endings are involved.

Fluid Resuscitation

Fluid resuscitation can be estimated using the Parkland formula (as listed in the following discussion) and is guided by hourly urine outputs. In children weighing 30 kg or less, urine output should be 1 mL per kilogram per hour; in adults, urine output should be 30 to 50 mL per hour. All patients with more than 20% total body surface area (TBSA) burns should have a Foley catheter and a nasogastric tube placed. Nasogastric tubes are placed to avoid aspiration secondary to burn ileus.

The following is the Parkland Formula:

24-hour fluid requirement = 4 mL × % TBSA burned × weight (kg)
1/2 volume given in first 8 hours
1/2 volume given over second 16 hours
(IV fluid should be lactated Ringer's solution.)

Other Treatment Considerations

Water evaporation is greatest in third-degree burns, so fluids must be monitored and adjusted according to urine output. Another initial consideration in burn patients is myoglobinuria, which should be recognized and treated to prevent renal failure. Treatment includes adequate IV hydration, mannitol diuresis, and alkalinization of the urine with bicarbonate.

Jewelry should be removed from burn patients to avoid a tourniquet effect when swelling occurs. Escharotomy, incision of the tight burned skin, may be required on deep circumferential extremity burns and the thorax. Distal pulses should be monitored by Doppler.

PEARL: Antibiotics are not indicated in the initial burn setting. Tetanus prophylaxis is required in all burn patients except those who have been actively immunized within the past 12 months.

WOUND CARE

Minor burns are initially treated with cold compresses followed by skin (blister) debridement and coverage with either a biologic dressing or topical antimicrobial.

CONTROVERSY: Some clinicians advocate leaving blisters intact to serve as a natural biologic dressing.

Large burns are debrided and treated with topical antimicrobials until excision and skin grafting takes

Table 25–1. COMMON ANTIMICROBIAL AGENTS USED FOR TREATMENT OF BURNS

Agent	Advantages	Disadvantages
Silver nitrate	Broad-spectrum, painless, no need for occlusive dressing	Nonpenetrating, electrolyte imbalances, stains everything black
Silver sulfadiazine (Silvadene)	Painless, no need for occlusive dressing; agent of choice for small burns	Lacks *Pseudomonas* coverage, little penetration, neutropenia
Mafenide (Sulfamylon)	Penetrates eschar; agent of choice for contaminated wounds	Poor *Staphylococcus* coverage, painful, some allergic reactions

place. Most burn centers advocate early excision and grafting. Table 25–1 lists the advantages and disadvantages of treatment with common antimicrobials.

With major burns, the reestablishment of skin integrity is a goal of therapy. Once the patient is stable and beyond the resuscitation phase, many centers perform burn wound excision with skin graft coverage. Many patients require multiple operations over several weeks to accomplish this goal.

Complications

Burn wound excision with skin grafting can be accompanied by significant blood loss. Major fluid shifts during these excision operations can result in a challenge for the anesthetist.

Infection is another worrisome complication of burns. Infection can convert a second-degree burn to a third-degree burn. The most common organism in burn wound infection is *Pseudomonas*. The reestablishment of skin integrity greatly minimizes the risks of infection.

REHABILITATION

Once skin integrity is accomplished, rehabilitation is begun. Rehabilitation is a team effort and may take months to accomplish fully.

Respiratory Failure and Ventilators

This chapter discusses the definition and classification of ARF (acute respiratory failure) and its management. Indications for instituting and weaning mechanical ventilation are also discussed. Respiratory failure can be acute or chronic. In surgical patients, it is almost always of the acute nature, and this is the focus of our discussion.

ACUTE RESPIRATORY FAILURE

The pulmonary system has two main functions: the oxygenation of blood and the elimination of carbon dioxide (CO_2). Either of these primary functions or a combination of both may fail and cause acute respiratory failure. **PEARL: Acute respiratory failure is characterized by either poor oxygenation (PaO_2 on room air ≤50), poor ventilation ($PaCO_2$≥50), or both.**

Pathophysiology

Types of ARF

When oxygenation fails such that PaO_2 on room air is 50 mm Hg or less, this is called type I or hypoxemic respiratory failure. Type I ARF is usually the result of a ventilation-perfusion ($\dot{V}/\dot{Q}$) mismatch. In the severest form of a $\dot{V}/\dot{Q}$ mismatch there is complete lack of ventilation to a segment of lung, resulting in a shunt, another cause of hypoxemia. Common clinical causes of type I ARF are listed in Table 26–1.

Type II or hypercapneic respiratory failure is characterized by the inability of the respiratory system to eliminate CO_2 and is characterized by a $PaCO_2$ of 50 mm Hg or more. It is caused by alveolar hypoventilation. Because an elevated $PaCO_2$ normally triggers an increased ventilatory drive, patients with type II ARF either are unable to sense the increased $PaCO_2$, are unable to signal increased ventilation, or lack the chest-lung function to increase ventilation. Common causes of type II ARF are listed in Table 26–1. **PEARL: The two most common causes of ARF on a surgical service are nosocomial pneumonia and adult respiratory distress syndrome (ARDS), both of which will be discussed further at the end of this chapter.**

Table 26–1. CAUSES OF ACUTE RESPIRATORY FAILURE

Type I (hypoxemic)

Infection: bacterial, viral, fungal, mycoplasma, other
Trauma: pulmonary contusion
Neoplasm
Other: bronchospasm, asthma, chronic obstructive
  pulmonary disease, heart failure, adult respiratory distress
  syndrome, pulmonary emboli, atelectasis, interstitial lung
  disease

Type II (hypercapneic)

Drugs: opioids, benzodiazepines, propofol, barbiturates
Metabolic: alkalosis, myxedema, hyponatremia
Neoplasm: brain tumor
Infection: meningitis, epiglottitis
Trauma: spinal cord injury, rib fractures, flail chest,
  pneumothorax
Other: increased intracranial pressure, vocal cord paralysis,
  laryngeal edema, pleural effusion, pain

Diagnosis

Symptoms

Common symptoms of ARF include the following:

- Abnormal respiratory rate (either high or low) or pattern
- Gasping and use of accessory muscles
- Cyanosis or diaphoresis
- Apprehension, restlessness, and distress
- Hypoxemia, often manifesting as alterations in mental status, tachycardia, and hypertension
- Hypercapnia, often manifesting as a depressed mental status (narcosis)

Clinical Findings

The diagnosis of ARF requires arterial blood gas (ABG) measurement and a chest x-ray.

Management

PEARL: During ARF, immediate considerations are reversal of life-threatening hypoxemia, hypercapnia, and acidosis (if present). This may require definitive diagnosis and immediate intervention directed toward the underlying problem (such as chest tube placement for a pneumothorax). Often, before a definitive diagnosis is reached, appropriate support for ARF must be instituted.

Patients whose respiratory compromise is not severe enough to require intubation may be managed by less invasive means.

Supplemental Oxygen

Supplemental oxygen can be provided by nasal cannula and by a variety of face masks.

- Oxygen by nasal cannula is regulated by increasing the flow rate (1 to 6 L/min). Each liter per minute of flow provides an additional 3 to 4% of inspired oxygen concentration (FiO_2). FiO_2 of up to about 45% can be provided, but the precise degree of supplementation is variable. This form of supplementation is recommended only for the mildest forms of respiratory distress.

- Venturi face masks are designed to provide higher levels of oxygen supplementation in a more accurate delivery system. Oxygen (100%) is pumped into the mask at high flow rates and the mask is designed to entrain room air through a valve that allows for a specific final FiO_2 that can be predetermined to be from 24% to about 60%.

- To achieve higher levels of FiO_2, face masks with oxygen reservoirs (small plastic bags) attached may be used. These are commonly referred to as 100% nonrebreather masks and can achieve FiO_2 of about 90%. Nonrebreather masks are useful to temporarily provide high levels of oxygen to a patient before endotracheal intubation.

Noninvasive Positive Pressure Ventilation

In noninvasive positive pressure ventilation, a specially designed, tightly fitting mask is placed over the patient's nose and mouth and is connected to a conventional ventilator. In this way, positive pressure breaths with increased oxygen concentrations can be provided.

CONTROVERSY: *Although occasionally helpful to buy time and avoid intubation while mild ARF resolves, positive pressure ventilation has many pitfalls and limitations. These include poor tolerance, tendency toward difficulty in clearing secretions, and forcing air into the stomach and GI tract.*

Pharmacologic Therapy

Several categories of medication are useful in the management of ARF, particularly that caused by obstructive airway diseases such as asthma and chronic obstructive pulmonary disease (COPD), and by pneumonia. These include:

- **β_2-agonists.** These drugs, delivered as aerosols and nebulizers into the airways, cause bronchial and smooth muscle relaxation. This group includes albuterol, metaproterenol, and terbutaline.

- **Anticholinergic agents.** Ipratropium, usually administered from a metered inhaler, causes bronchial smooth muscle relaxation. These agents are not as fast-acting as β_2-agonists.
- **Corticosteroids.** Methylprednisolone (IV) and prednisone (oral) are commonly used for severe asthma and COPD exacerbations. Their mechanism of action is anti-inflammatory in nature.
- **Theophylline preparations.** IV aminophylline, administered as a continuous infusion, is an important bronchodilator that is often used in ARF due to obstructive airway disease. It requires careful monitoring of serum levels to maximize efficacy and avoid side effects.
- **Antibiotics.** These drugs are necessary for the management of pneumonia. On a surgical service, we most commonly see nosocomial pneumonias as a cause of ARF (see Nosocomial Pneumonia later in this chapter).

ENDOTRACHEAL INTUBATION AND VENTILATORY SUPPORT

Indications

The indications for intubation and ventilatory support mirror the causes of ARF as previously described. It is common to use criteria to assist in the decision to intubate and ventilate, but these criteria are not fixed in stone. Therefore, a good clinical assessment remains important. Patients who are clinically deteriorating from a known clinical condition might need to be intubated before criteria are met. Conversely, a patient may avoid intubation despite meeting criteria if the clinical situation is expected to resolve quickly and the patient has adequate reserve.

Specific criteria for intubation and ventilation include the following:

- Inadequate oxygenation
  - PaO_2 <55 mm Hg on room air
  - PaO_2 <70 mm Hg on 50% face mask
- Inadequate ventilation
  - $PaCO_2$ >60 mm Hg
  - pH <7.25

Orotracheal versus Nasotracheal Intubation

Orotracheal intubation is more common because it is technically easier to perform than nasotracheal intubation, particularly in emergency conditions. However, nasotracheal intubation offers the advantage of better patient comfort, particularly if a lengthy intubation is expected. Nasotracheal intubation is best performed in a spontaneously breathing patient and may require use of a smaller-sized endotracheal tube. If a patient remains on ventilatory support with endotracheal intubation for a lengthy period of time (e.g., 2 to 3 weeks), conversion to a tracheostomy is recommended. In this setting, a tracheostomy offers better patient comfort, allows for easier tracheal suctioning, and likely promotes weaning from ventilatory support.

MECHANICAL VENTILATORS

A variety of ventilators are available and commonly used, but the specific names and models are not important. It is important that all are capable of being set to accommodate the needs of virtually any patient. You need to become familiar with the model or models that your hospital uses.

PEARL: The best way to learn about a given ventilator is not to be intimidated and to ask a respiratory therapist to give you a tour of the ventilator and its major settings. Ventilators provide breaths (cycle) to patients either in a predetermined or set volume (volume-cycled) or up to a predetermined or set pressure (pressure-cycled). For adults, volume-cycled ventilators are by far the most common.

Modes of Mechanical Ventilation

PEARL: The major modes of ventilatory support are Intermittent Mandatory Ventilation (IMV) and Assist Control (AC). Each has many variations.

Intermittent Mandatory Ventilation (IMV)

In IMV (often called synchronized or SIMV), the ventilator delivers a predetermined tidal volume (V_T) a preset number of times each minute. Tidal volumes are set at 8 to 10 mL/kg or usually between 600 and 750 mL for average-sized adults. Rates usually vary from 2 to 20, depending on the patient's needs. What distinguishes SIMV from AC is that when the patient initiates his or her own breath, the ventilator does not assist in the breath, and the tidal volume of the breath is dependent on how hard the patient breathes (i.e., the more negative inspiratory force the patient uses, the larger the V_T). Therefore, the patient must exert energy and work to obtain breaths above the ventilator's set rate. This mode is often used while the patient's ARF is resolving as a means of gradually allowing the patient to assume more of the work of breathing and wean from ventilatory support.

Assist Control (AC)

In AC mode, the rate and tidal volume are also set, but any time the patient breathes or triggers the ventilator (generates a small, negative inspiratory force), it delivers a full tidal volume breath. In this way, the patient does not work very hard to be ventilated above the set rate. This mode is often used when ventilatory support is initiated because it provides maximum support.

Adjuncts to Ventilatory Support

Several adjuncts to ventilatory support can be applied in either SIMV or AC mode, such as positive end–expiratory pressure (PEEP), pressure support, and continuous positive airway pressure (CPAP). **PEARL: PEEP, often used in patients with ARDS, can be applied to prevent airway pressure from falling below a set amount (5 to 20 cm H_2O) at the end of expiration; this prevents end expiratory alveolar collapse, maintains functional residual capacity (FRC), and promotes better oxygenation.** Many practitioners use physiologic levels of PEEP (5 cm H_2O) on all patients with an endotracheal tube.

- **PEEP.** Higher levels of PEEP are most commonly used in ARDS to decrease the intrapulmonary shunt and thereby increase oxygenation and decrease FiO_2 requirements. The major disadvantages of PEEP, particularly at higher levels, are mild hemodynamic compromise (i.e., decreased blood pressure, decreased cardiac output) and an increased incidence of barotrauma (pneumothorax).
- **Pressure support.** Here, the patient's spontaneous inspirations are enhanced by added pressure. This helps the patient overcome any increased resistance and work of breathing that result from the disease process and the mechanics of the ventilator and endotracheal tube. This can promote better patient-ventilator interaction, particularly during the weaning process.
- **CPAP** provides an elevated baseline pressure for all breaths and is therefore equivalent to PEEP plus pressure support. It is useful in many forms of ARF to increase FRC, improve compliance, and enhance gas exchange.

What Needs to Be Set and How to Decide What's Best for Your Patient

A number of parameters need to be specified when a patient is receiving ventilatory support. In addition to the ventilatory mode (IMV or AC), ventilatory parameters and goals needs to be specified, as listed in Table 26–2.

Although most patients are extubated in the operating room at the conclusion of their operation, some are not for various reasons. Clinician preferences for the mode and details of ventilatory support vary widely. However, some guidelines and generalizations are worth mentioning:

- For a patient who is coming out of the operating room intubated and on ventilatory support, use AC mode at a rate of about 14 to 20 breaths per minute as long as the patient is still sedated.
- If the patient is more awake or begins to awaken and to initiate spontaneous respirations, begin to wean the patient from ventilatory support by switching to an IMV mode and gradually decreas-

Table 26–2. GOALS AND PARAMETERS OF VENTILATOR USE

Ventilatory Parameter	Setting	Goal
Mode	IMV or AC	To maintain patient comfort and synchrony with ventilator
FiO_2	40–100%	To maintain $PaO_2 >$ 80, oxygen saturation > 92%)
V_T	8–12 mL/kg	To maintain normal $PaCO_2$
Rate	2–20 breaths per minute	To maintain normal $PaCO_2$
PEEP	0 or 5 cm H_2O initially	To maintain FRC and improve oxygenation
Adjuncts	Pressure support or CPAP as needed	To maintain/improve oxygenation, decrease work of breathing

ing the rate so that the patient is forced to assume much of the work of breathing. This serves to assess the patient's ability to maintain adequate ventilatory function when extubated.

- If the patient is being treated for worsening ARF, an IMV mode is preferable so that muscles of respiration are continually used. If IMV is not tolerated, an AC mode is acceptable. Such patients often require higher levels of FiO_2 to maintain adequate oxygenation as well as PEEP or other pressure-supportive techniques.

- For patients who are emergently intubated, it is always wise to begin with 100% oxygen and titrate down as tolerated.

WEANING FROM MECHANICAL VENTILATION

As resolution of the patient's respiratory failure occurs, weaning from mechanical ventilation usually takes place on the IMV mode. **PEARL: A prerequisite to begin weaning from mechanical ventilation is a patient who is awake, alert, and able to follow commands.** Following are steps in the process of weaning a patient from mechanical ventilation:

- The preset ventilatory rate is incrementally decreased by 2 breaths per minute as the patient assumes a greater fraction of ventilation and work of breathing.
- During the incremental rate reduction, patients are monitored (clinically, with pulse oximetry, and arterial blood gases) to make certain that goals of ventilation and oxygenation are being met.
- The patient must be on no more than 40% O_2, 5 cm H_2O of PEEP, or 8 cm H_2O of pressure support.
- The addition of pressure support can sometimes facilitate the weaning process by overcoming the added resistance that is created by breathing through the ventilator circuit.
- When the patient is weaned to a rate of 2 to 6 breaths per minute, a series of mechanical weaning parameters (extubation criteria) are checked, which, if met, usually indicate that a patient will tolerate removal of support and extubation.

Extubation criteria are listed in Table 26–3.

If these criteria are met, many clinicians place the patient on T-bar (often called blow-by). This eliminates ventilator-initiated breaths but continues oxygen flow. T-bar placement should be done only for a short period (30 minutes) during which a final assessment (often including an ABG) is made before extubation. Many patients do not require this step. A patient who is doing

Table 26–3. EXTUBATION CRITERIA

NIF (negative inspiratory force)	$\leq$–25 cm H_2O
V_T (patient-generated tidal volume)	$\geq$5–6 mL/kg
Respiratory rate	10–25
Vital capacity	$\geq$10–15 mL/kg
Minute ventilation	$\leq$10–12 L/min

well can be extubated directly from a low IMV rate. Once extubated, the patient should immediately be placed on an oxygen mask (40% to 50%) to ensure adequate oxygenation. Depending on the clinical situation, an ABG is obtained about 30 minutes after extubation to ensure normal values. Oxygen support can be weaned to nasal cannula oxygen and eventually room air when clinically appropriate.

COMMON CAUSES OF ARF

Nosocomial Pneumonia

Nosocomial pneumonia is a pneumonia that develops in a hospitalized patient and is not community acquired. It is currently the second most common nosocomial infection, but carries the highest mortality of all nosocomial infections.

An important pathogenic mechanism of nosocomial pneumonia is believed to be colonization of the stomach and oropharynx with gram-negative enteric organisms (possibly fostered by stress gastritis prophylaxis with anti-acid medications) and their subsequent tracheal aspiration. Common organisms include *Pseudomonas, Klebsiella, Escherichia coli,* and *Enterobacter* species.

Risk factors for the development of nosocomial pneumonia include the following:

- General anesthesia
- Major abdominal or thoracic surgery
- Bed rest or immobilization
- Endotracheal intubation with ventilatory support

Signs and symptoms of nosocomial pneumonia can include the following:

- Productive cough
- Fever
- Leukocytosis
- Dyspnea
- Tachypnea
- Shortness of breath
- Hypoxemia

- Infiltrate on chest x-ray
- Sputum or endotracheal aspirate positive for white blood cells and bacteria
- Increasing ventilatory support requirements

Treatment

Treatment of nosocomial pneumonia includes IV antibiotics for 7 to 14 days and increased pulmonary toilet. Empiric antibiotic coverage with an extended-spectrum penicillin (e.g., piperacillin) and an aminoglycoside (e.g., tobramycin) is usually recommended. This double-drug regimen is favored because of the predominance of *Pseudomonas* as an offending organism. Single-drug regimens without an aminoglycoside may be suitable for patients with renal insufficiency and when *Pseudomonas* is not cultured. Antibiotics are often tailored further based on the culture and sensitivity data.

Adult Respiratory Distress Syndrome

The adult respiratory distress syndrome (ARDS) is a form of ARF of unclear etiology characterized by noncardiogenic pulmonary edema. The syndrome typically develops 24 to 72 hours after critical illnesses such as sepsis and multiple trauma. Diagnostic criteria for ARDS include the rapid onset of respiratory failure; development of new, diffuse, bilateral chest x-ray infiltrates; the absence of elevated cardiac filling pressures; decreased lung compliance; and a preexisting clinical condition (e.g., sepsis, multiple trauma, multiple blood transfusions) known to be a risk factor for ARDS.

The pathophysiology of ARDS includes injury to the pulmonary alveolar-capillary membrane, resulting in increased permeability, increased pulmonary vascular resistance, decreased pulmonary compliance, and increased intrapulmonary shunting. The activation of endogenous inflammatory processes (e.g., cytokines, complement, neutrophils, macrophages) is thought to be an important initiating factor.

Treatment

Treatment consists of maximally addressing the underlying clinical cause and providing ventilatory support, usually with increased positive end-expiratory pressures (PEEP) as needed. Despite these measures, the mortality rate averages 50% for all patients with ARDS and can be as high as 90% in certain patient groups particularly when other organ systems fail.

27
CHAPTER

Nutrition

Surgical patients frequently require nutritional support for preexisting malnutrition or for prevention of malnutrition during surgical or other stress states when they temporarily are unable to eat. To achieve these goals, an understanding of nutritional support and the best ways to provide such support is essential.

NUTRITIONAL ASSESSMENT

Subjective Global Assessment

PEARL: A subjective global assessment, consisting of a history and physical exam, is the best and simplest method of assessing a patient's nutritional status. Such a global assessment will be as accurate and much quicker and cheaper than any number of more sophisticated laboratory or other measurements.

The history should include the following information:

- Any decreased oral intake
- Weight loss
- Underlying disease
- Functional status of the patient

The physical exam primarily focuses on the presence of signs of weight loss and wasting:

- **Significant weight loss** is loss of 10% or more of body weight and signifies mild to moderate malnutrition.

- **Severe malnutrition** is weight loss of 20% or more of body weight.

A history of weight loss at these levels, along with a physical exam that corroborates weight loss, is very strong evidence that the patient will be at significant nutritional risk in a surgical stress setting and that nutritional support is likely indicated.

Supporting Evidence of Nutritional Status

Additional evidence to support the assessment of a patient's nutritional status relies on several other indicators. These indicators, although more sophisticated and costly, may provide a quantifiable nutritional assessment that allows the effects of therapy to be monitored.

Anthropomorphic Measurements

Anthropomorphic measurements include height, weight, skinfold thickness, and muscle circumference. These measurements are of limited practical value.

Biochemical Indicators of Malnutrition

Albumin level is useful in the initial assessment of patients who have chronic diseases and are in a steady state. In general, an albumin level of less than 3.0 g/dL is an indicator of malnutrition. Adequate nutritional status can be inferred from an albumin level of more than 3.5 g/dL.

PEARL: Because of the long half-life of albumin—21 days— and its distribution in the extravascular space, albumin level has little value as a short-term index of nutrition during acute illness.

Rapid turnover proteins include transferrin (half-life 8 days; less than 200 mg/dL suggests malnutrition), thyroxin-binding prealbumin (half-life 2 days), and retinol-binding protein (half-life 12 hours). These proteins are made in the liver and, because of their short half-lives, are better indicators than albumin of acute nutritional depletion. They are also useful in following a patient's response to nutritional supplementation.

Immune Function

Because the immune system and its proper function are dependent on nutritional status, certain immune parameters can be used to assess nutritional status:

- A total lymphocyte count of less than 1200 cells/mm^3 (calculated from total white blood cell [WBC] count multiplied by % lymphocytes) indicates malnutrition.
- Loss of delayed cutaneous hypersensitivity (anergy), assessed by skin testing, is a sign of malnutrition. This is of limited clinical value in an acute setting owing to difficulties with its standardized measurement and the prevalence of confounding immunocompromised states.

Nitrogen Balance

A state of nitrogen loss is associated with malnutrition. Nitrogen balance measurements are useful to follow a hospitalized patient's response to nutritional support. It requires a 24-hour urine collection and is calculated using the following equations.

Nitrogen balance = Nitrogen intake − Nitrogen output
Nitrogen intake = (g protein over 24 hrs)/6.25
Nitrogen output = 24-hour urinary urea nitrogen (UUN, g/day) + (UUN × 0.2) + 2

NUTRITIONAL REQUIREMENTS

PEARL: Caloric needs for average patients are 25 to 30 kcal/kg per day; protein needs are 1.0 g/kg per day. Caloric needs are therefore about 2000 kcal per day for an average 70-kg patient. For stressed patients, particularly those with critical illness, caloric needs are increased to 35 to 40 kcal/kg per day, and protein needs are increased to 1.5 g/kg per day. Carbohydrates are the predominant caloric source. Fat provides about 20 to 30 percent of the total caloric input.

Specific individual needs can also be calculated using the Harris-Benedict equations. These equations (too complicated to be listed here; see your hospital's nutritionist or consult a more detailed surgical text), based on the patient's sex, weight, height, and age, determine **basal energy expenditure** (BEE).

Patients in a hospital are rarely in a basal state and have increased caloric needs because of stress and illness. These increased needs can be estimated as anywhere from 20 to 110 percent above the BEE, depending on the nature of the illness. For example, caloric needs are increased under the following conditions:

- By 20% in minor surgery
- By 35% in major skeletal trauma
- By 60% in major sepsis
- By 110% in major burns

Indirect calorimetry can be used to measure a patient's oxygen consumption and carbon dioxide production, from which energy expenditure in calories can be calculated. This is a fairly sophisticated, labor-intensive, and user-dependent technique, in which a patient breathes into a machine for 30 to 60 minutes, and gases are then analyzed to provide the measurements. Indirect calorimetry can also be used to calculate a **respiratory quotient** (RQ), which provides an index of the mixture of fuel utilization and is helpful in adjusting nutritional support.

CONTROVERSY: Data from indirect calorimetry must be interpreted cautiously, because it represents a "snapshot" determination and is subject to variability.

INDICATIONS FOR NUTRITIONAL SUPPORT

Indications for nutritional support are varied and quite controversial. Absolute indications for nutritional support include patients who cannot achieve an adequate oral intake (e.g., those with stroke, dementia, or esophageal obstruction) and those who have a non-functioning gastrointestinal (GI) tract (e.g., severe postoperative ileus or short bowel syndrome).

In the management of acute surgical diseases, the indications for nutritional support are less clear. In the following sections we will discuss the types of patients on a surgical service that benefit from nutritional support.

Preoperative Nutritional Support

Patients who are undergoing major abdominal or thoracic surgery for management of cancer are often malnourished preoperatively and would not be expected to recover GI tract function for several days or longer after surgery. **PEARL: Preoperative nutritional support is of value in patients who have severe malnutrition (i.e., loss of more than 10% of body weight and an albumin level of less than 3).** In these patients, studies indicate that preoperative nutritional support (enteral or parenteral), for 7 to 10 days preoperatively and until bowel function and oral diet are resumed postoperatively, decreases morbidity and mortality. This benefit has not been shown for patients who are mildly or moderately malnourished.

(In these studies, the degree of malnutrition was calculated using nutritional indicators, thus allowing stratification of the patients.)

Postoperative Nutritional Support

Starvation in the postoperative setting for up to 7 to 10 days is well tolerated and without significant sequelae. Usually, diet is resumed within several days after elective surgery, and nutritional support is rarely required. **PEARL: Elderly patients, with less nutritional reserve than younger patients, may require nutritional support by postoperative day 5 to 7 if diet has not resumed.**

Surgical Diseases That Often Require Nutritional Support

There are several conditions for which nutritional support, by the enteral or parenteral route, is commonly provided, including the following:

- Prolonged postoperative ileus
- Severe acute pancreatitis
- Major trauma and burns
- Enterocutaneous fistula

ENTERAL NUTRITION

There are two varieties of nutritional support: **enteral** (via the gut) and **parenteral** (via an intravenous route). When nutritional support is deemed necessary and the GI tract is functional, enteral nutrition is indicated. **PEARL: Enteral nutrition is preferred over parenteral nutrition. (If the gut works, use it.)** Parenteral nutrition should be used only if enteral nutrition is not possible or has failed.

Depending on the needs of the patient, enteral nutrition can be supplied via several routes, often dictated by the patient's condition and the expected duration of support.

Methods of Short-Term Supplementation

Oral

Products such as Ensure and Sustacal can be drunk out of the can and provide 1 kcal/mL; each can contains 240 mL.

Nasogastric Tube

A small-bore, Dobhoff-like tube is inserted through the nose into the stomach. After placement, tube position should be confirmed by aspirating gastric contents, and by injecting air and hearing it through a stethoscope placed over the stomach. Finally, an x-ray is taken for confirmation. **PEARL: Tube placement is checked in several different ways to ensure that the tube has not been placed into the tracheobronchial tree and that it extends beyond the esophagus and well into the stomach.** Patients getting nasogastric feedings should not have a history of reflux or known aspiration pneumonia and ideally should be kept in as upright a position as possible to avoid reflux and aspiration.

Rate and Type of Feeding

Feedings should be initiated at a continuous rate of about 25 mL per hour. Gastric residuals should be measured periodically to confirm that feedings are not accumulating in the stomach, which might indicate poor tolerance and risk for aspiration. A residual of up to twice the infused rate is usually acceptable. The rate of feeds is advanced by 25 mL per hour each day until the target needs (usually 85 to 100 mL/hr) are met.

An alternative is **bolus feeding,** which is given as 200 to 400 mL per bolus every 4 hours. Bolus feeding is easier on nursing staff or family and eliminates the need for a continuous-infusion pump. However, risks of aspiration may be increased, so we recommend that patients first prove that they can tolerate continuous feeds before switching to bolus feeds.

Strength of Feeding

Because the stomach is normally capable of handling hyperosmolar food, isosmolar tube feeds (as most are) can be given at full strength. Hyperosmolar food products can be started at half strength and then advanced to full strength if tolerated. Tube maintenance is important; the tube should be flushed with water once or twice a day.

Nasointestinal Tube

A nasointestinal tube is a small-bore tube that is passed through the nose and ends up in the duodenum (or even the proximal jejunum). It may reach the duodenum by normal peristalsis (often aided by metoclopramide and patient positioning), or it may be guided into the duodenum under fluoroscopy or with the aid of endoscopy. In patients with reflux or gastric hypomotility or atony (as may occur after a major abdominal operation), duodenal feeds are often tolerated. **PEARL: Because the duodenum normally handles only isosmolar food, hyperosmolar food products should be diluted initially when administered via a nasoduodenal tube.** Often, after some acclimatization, the concentration can be increased.

Jejunostomy Tube

Sometimes during major abdominal surgery, a feeding **jejunostomy** tube is surgically placed into the proximal jejunum to provide early postoperative enteral nutrition. The tube exits directly through the abdominal wall. A wide variety of tubes may be used. The tube usually can be easily removed shortly after surgery if the patient resumes oral feeding, or it may be left in place for continued or supplemental feedings if deemed necessary.

The advantage of the jejunostomy tube is its ability to provide enteral nutrition to the small bowel almost immediately after major abdominal surgery despite the perceived ileus.

Methods of Long-Term Supplementation

Gastrostomy Tube

A **gastrostomy** tube is a tube placed through the skin of the abdominal wall directly into the stomach. Placement can be by open surgical technique or, more commonly, by a less invasive technique, such as **percutaneous endoscopic gastrostomy** (PEG). The advantage of PEG is that it eliminates the need for open abdominal surgery and its required anesthetic. The most common candidates for gastrostomy tubes include:

- Patients with dementia or strokes who are unable to eat or swallow
- Patients who have undergone major head and neck surgery that precludes adequate swallowing
- Patients being treated for various malignancies who need to supplement nutritional intake

Prerequisites for gastrostomy tube placement include documentation of adequate gastric emptying and absence of reflux. Gastrostomy tubes are suitable for both continuous and bolus feeds with any enteral product, including foods processed in a blender.

Jejunostomy Tube

If long-term feeds are required and placement of a gastrostomy tube is contraindicated (e.g., patient has known reflux or history of aspiration pneumonia), a feeding jejunostomy tube may be surgically placed. Placement requires an open surgical procedure and carries significant morbidity and even mortality, owing to the malnourished state and concomitant conditions from which these patients suffer. Continuous infusion of isosmolar enteral products with the jejunostomy tube is the norm.

Enteral Supplementation Products

A multitude of products are available for enteral nutritional support, but the simplest and least expensive products are best. The complex and specialized products are expensive and should be used only if clearly indicated. Enteral products can best be summarized in the following categories:

- **Oral supplements.** These are flavored products designed to be taken by mouth. Examples are Ensure, Sustacal, and Carnation Instant Breakfast.
- **Tube feeding products.** These products are designed to be administered through feeding tubes and there are several categories.

  - **Polymeric products.** These contain a complete diet with intact protein (e.g., they require intraluminal digestion). Polymeric products are usually lactose-free, contain 1 kcal/mL, and are isosmolar. Examples are Osmolite and Isocal.
  - **High–caloric-density products.** These provide a complete diet with intact protein, contain up to 2 kcal/mL, and are hyperosmolar (must be given into the stomach or diluted if given directly into the small bowel). High–caloric-density products are indicated in patients with increased caloric needs (e.g., major burns) and volume restrictions (e.g., congestive heart failure). An example is Magnacal.
  - **Monomeric products.** These products contain elemental nutrients (e.g., protein as amino acids or small peptides) that require little to no intraluminal digestion (i.e., just absorption), are low-residue, and are usually hyperosmolar. Examples are Vivonex and Criticare.

Complications of Enteral Nutritional Support

The following are complications that may result from enteral nutritional support:

- **Aspiration pneumonia.** The best treatment is prevention.
- **Feeding intolerance.** This manifests as vomiting, distention, and cramping. After an ileus is ruled out, try slowing the rate or diluting the product.
- **Diarrhea.** Rule out other causes (e.g., *Clostridium difficile* colitis). Treat by diluting hyperosmolar products or adding antidiarrheal agents (kaolin and pectin, psyllium, diphenoxylate-atropine sulfate, loperamide).
- **Metabolic complications.** Hyperglycemia and hyperosmotic nonketotic coma (rare) are possible complications.

PARENTERAL NUTRITION

Parenteral nutrition, also called **total parenteral nutrition** (TPN) or nutrition by vein, is indicated when the enteral route is not possible or has been tried and failed. TPN should always be considered as a second line of nutritional support, because it is significantly more complicated and more costly, involves more risks and complications, and is much less physiologic than enteral nutrition. Clinical conditions that usually require TPN include:

- Gastrointestinal fistulas
- Short bowel syndrome
- Major burns with ileus
- Radiation enteritis
- Acute GI toxicity due to chemotherapy
- Severe pancreatitis
- Prolonged ileus

Composition

TPN provides nutrition in a solution consisting of dextrose (carbohydrate) and amino acids (protein), supplemented by a lipid emulsion (fat), which is administered through a central vein. The final dextrose concentration is usually 20 or 25%, and the amino acid final concentration is about 5%. This provides about 1 kcal/mL of nonprotein calories. The solution also contains basic electrolytes (Na^+, Cl^-, K^+), minerals and trace elements (e.g., zinc, copper), vitamins, and occasionally certain additives (insulin, cimetidine). Fat calories are provided by a 10 or 20% lipid emulsion, which is usually piggybacked into the central line or occasionally mixed directly in. **PEARL: A standard TPN regimen is 20% dextrose (D_{20}) with 5% amino acids at 80 to 100 mL/hr, with lipids given twice weekly. This provides about 2000 kcal per day.**

Administration

Because of the high dextrose concentration and high osmolality of parenteral solutions, TPN must be administered into a large vein with large blood flow. Suitable sites include:

- The superior vena cava via a central line placed into the subclavian or internal jugular vein
- The inferior vena cava via a line placed into the femoral vein (less preferable due to increased infectious and thrombotic complications)

An alternative site is a **peripherally inserted central catheter** (PICC) line placed through an arm vein and threaded through the subclavian vein and into the superior vena cava, which avoids central venous puncture.

PEARL: Central line placement for TPN is ideally placed in a well-hydrated patient under controlled conditions. Significant coagulopathy should be treated. Central line placement must take place according to established guidelines and under strict sterile conditions. A chest x-ray is obtained to confirm line location and to rule out pneumothorax.

To avoid hyperglycemia, TPN must be started at about 40 mL per hour for the first day and the rate increased by 20 to 40 mL per hour per day. The rate is increased until the target rate, based on the patient's nutritional needs, is reached (usually about 2 to 3 days).

Monitoring

Patients on TPN require significant monitoring of the following parameters to optimize the therapy and avoid complications:

- Vital signs are taken at every shift.
- Glucose fingersticks are required once or twice daily, along with serum confirmation about twice weekly.
- Twenty-four-hour fluid input and output measurements are taken.
- Blood work should be performed at least twice weekly for electrolytes, glucose, liver function tests, calcium, and phosphorus, and weekly for PT/PTT (prothrombin time/partial thromboplastin time) and short-turnover proteins.
- Weight should be checked once or twice weekly.

TPN Formulations

A number of different TPN formulations are available to meet the special nutritional needs of various disease states:

- **Standard.** D_{20} or D_{25} with 4 to 6% amino acids with lipids two to three times per week.
- **Stress.** D_{15} (to decrease calorie to nitrogen ratio requirements and glucose intolerance in critical illness) with 5 to 6% amino acids (to meet increased protein requirements) enriched with branched-chain amino acids (preferentially used in critical illness), and daily lipids (to meet increased caloric requirements). This formulation is indicated for hypermetabolic, traumatized, and septic patients.
- **Renal.** D_{50} (to increase caloric density and reduce fluid requirements) with 2% amino acids (to decrease protein load in order to prevent rise in blood urea nitrogen and therefore delay or prevent dialysis) and low electrolytes. This formulation is indicated in acute renal failure.
- **Cardiac.** D_{50} (to increase caloric density and reduce fluid requirements) with 4 to 6% amino acids. This formulation is indicated for patients with congestive heart failure.

- **Hepatic.** D_{20} or D_{25} with 3.5% amino acids (to prevent protein intolerance with hepatic failure) enriched with branched-chain amino acids. Aromatic amino acids, which may serve as false neurotransmitters, are reduced. This formulation is indicated for patients with hepatic failure and encephalopathy.

Complications

TPN has many potential complications. Early technical complications (related to line placement) include:

- Pneumothorax
- Hemothorax due to lacerating subclavian vein or hitting subclavian artery
- Brachial plexus injury
- Thoracic duct injury (on left side only)
- Catheter embolus
- Air embolus
- Catheter malposition (that is, up neck or across to other side)

Late technical complications include:

- Septic complications—central line sepsis (in about 2 to 10%). It is manifested by systemic infection due to colonization of the catheter with bacteria, leading to bacteremia. If recognized early, sepsis can often be treated by removal of the catheter. For significant systemic signs of infection, antibiotics (usually vancomycin to cover gram-positive staphylococcal species) are recommended in addition to catheter removal.
- Subclavian vein thrombosis

Metabolic complications include:

- Hyperglycemia. Treat with insulin in TPN, usually starting with 10 units regular insulin per liter and titrating to maintain glucose between 150 and 200.

PEARL: Sudden unexplained hyperglycemia in a patient who had previously been tolerating TPN should alert one to the possibility of an infection, with line sepsis being high on the differential.

- Hypoglycemia, usually related to increased insulin doses in the TPN or sudden cessation of TPN. If TPN is accidentally stopped suddenly, an IV solution of D_5 or D_{10} is sufficient to stop this complication.
- Liver dysfunction, usually due to increased fat storage in hepatocytes, often manifested as increased alkaline phosphatase and bilirubin. It is best managed by decreasing the dextrose concentration of the TPN to no more than D_{15}.

28

CHAPTER

Patient Monitoring in the ICU

The surgical intensive care unit (SICU) can be an intimidating environment to medical students and junior residents. The complexity of surgical critical illness and the concomitant complexity of its care present a challenge to those not well acquainted with critical care. This chapter introduces you to the many ways patients are monitored in an ICU so that you can become familiar with the language of critical care and the advanced technology commonly used.

ROUTINE VITAL SIGNS

Monitoring a patient's physical exam as frequently as is necessary is foremost in the care of critically ill patients. **PEARL: The patient's physical exam should never be ignored, no matter how sophisticated the monitoring devices are.**

The basic vital signs include:

- Heart rate (HR)
- Blood pressure (BP)
- Respiratory rate (RR)
- Temperature

PEARL: A patient with an HR of over 100 or a systolic BP below 90 is classified as hemodynamically unstable.

Such vital signs require immediate and unrelenting attention until a presumptive cause is found and therapy has been implemented. The physician should get into the habit of looking at trends rather than single values.

A *decreased* RR may be a manifestation of oversedation. An *increased* RR may be a sign of increased anxiety, pain, or impending and early respiratory failure, despite a normal PaO_2. An increased temperature is a common sign of infection, but hypothermia occasionally occurs in profoundly septic patients.

FLUID BALANCE

Intake and Output (I and O)

Careful attention to fluid balance requires tabulation of a patient's intake and output and determination of the balance. In a normal patient, fluid balance should result in a positive value of about 500 to 1000 mL. This is due to **insensible losses** (mostly respiratory) that cannot be measured or included in the balance calculation. Patients with critical illness tend to have higher insensible losses owing to mechanical ventilation, elevated temperature, or both. In addition, many critical illnesses (sepsis, trauma, immediate postop period) result in increased third-space losses (ileus, edema, intraperitoneal inflammation), thus further exaggerating the net positive balance.

PEARL: A positive value higher than 1500 mL should prompt further investigation. Persistently elevated positive fluid balance should prompt attempts at limiting fluid intake or inducing diuresis, if appropriate.

Weight

Another practical gauge of overall fluid balance is change in body weight. In the acute setting, weight change is caused by fluid gain or loss. Unfortunately, accurate measurement of body weight in ICU patients is difficult.

PULSE OXIMETRY

Pulse oximeters are noninvasive devices that allow estimation of hemoglobin oxygen saturation (SaO_2) through the skin by measuring the color (or light absorbance) of blood. This correlates with the fraction of oxygenated and deoxygenated hemoglobin. They also provide pulse rate. Pulse oximeters are applied to the fingertips, ear lobes, or toes. They have become universally used in ICUs and many other hospital settings.

Although pulse oximeters provide very valuable information, a number of caveats or pitfalls must be kept in mind:

- An arterial-like waveform that correlates with the patient's pulse must be visible on the screen.
- Significant PaO_2 drops (e.g., from 100 to the 60s) accompany smaller decreases in SaO_2 (from 100 to 90%). Such changes may have significant clinical or diagnostic implications, and correlation with arterial blood gases (ABGs) is necessary in many situations.
- Adequate ventilation cannot be assumed based on oximetric data only.
- Measurement is unreliable in settings of poor tissue perfusion states (e.g., shock), hypothermia, and the use of vasopressor drugs.

ARTERIAL LINES

Arterial lines are small catheters inserted into arteries for the purpose of monitoring BP and allowing frequent arterial blood sampling for ABG and other lab value determinations. They are used under the following conditions:

- Patients with respiratory failure, to follow their ABGs while they are on ventilatory support
- Patients with shock states or hemodynamic instability, particularly if vasoactive drugs are being used to closely monitor BP

The arterial catheter is connected to a monitor via liquid-filled tubing and a transducer so that an arterial waveform and measurements of systolic, diastolic, and mean arterial BP are displayed on the monitor.

Sites

PEARL: Arterial lines are placed, in order of preference, in the radial, femoral, axillary and dorsalis pedis arteries. The brachial artery should be avoided as a site because of poor collateral circulation and a higher complication rate. The radial artery is far and away the most common and preferred site because of the dual blood supply of the hand and because of patient ease. **PEARL: An Allen's test should always be performed to confirm patency of the ulnar artery and palmar arch and the ability of the ulnar artery to perfuse the hand in the event of radial artery thrombosis (Table 28–1).**

Complications

The following are complications, generally uncommon, resulting from arterial lines:

- Infection (line sepsis)
- Hematoma
- Distal ischemia
- Arterial thrombosis
- Pseudoaneurysm formation

To prevent infection, arterial lines should be placed under full sterile technique and maintained under an

Table 28–1. ALLEN'S TEST

1. With the patient's fingertips facing you and with the palm up, use the second and third fingers of both of your hands to occlude the radial and ulnar pulses by grasping tightly around both sides of the wrist.
2. Have the patient close and open his or her hand several times to exsanguinate blood from the hand and give it a white, blanched appearance.
3. While watching the open hand, release the ulnar artery while maintaining pressure on the radial artery, and watch the reperfusion (pinking up) of the radial half of the hand.
4. A positive test is elicited when it takes more than 5 seconds for the radial side of the hand to pink-up. If positive, another arterial site (other hand or different site) should be selected for cannulation.

occlusive (usually transparent) sterile dressing. **PEARL: The catheter for the arterial line should be changed when indicated by signs of infection at the site or systemic bacteremia when another source cannot be identified.**

The extremity that contains an arterial line should always be monitored for signs of distal ischemia, and, if it is present, the line should be promptly removed. Vascular surgery consultation should be obtained if ischemic signs persist after catheter removal.

CENTRAL VENOUS CATHETERS

Central venous pressure (CVP) catheters, commonly called central lines, are catheters inserted percutaneously into the subclavian and internal jugular veins and advanced into the superior vena cava. These catheters are about 8 inches long and have up to three lumens at their end. They are inserted using a guidewire-through-needle technique (Seldinger technique). The following are clinical indications for the use of CVP catheters:

- For optimal venous access (e.g., because of poor peripheral venous access, need for high-volume fluid resuscitation, administration of vasoactive drugs)
- For the administration of total parenteral nutrition
- For monitoring CVP

When CVP lines are hooked up to transducers, they allow measurement of CVP. This is equivalent to right atrial pressure and provides an index of the heart's preload status (i.e., filling pressure), which is a determinant of cardiac output.

Occasionally, determination of the CVP is helpful in the management of a patient with hypotension or low urine output because a low CVP suggests volume depletion and a high CVP suggests congestive heart failure. In fact, in healthy hearts there is a good correlation between right-heart CVP and left-heart preload. **PEARL: In many critically ill patients with cardiac and pulmonary dysfunction, CVP is not an accurate assessment of left-heart preload status. A more accurate assessment often requires insertion of a pulmonary artery catheter.**

Complications of CVP lines are early ones related to their insertion (e.g., pneumothorax and hemothorax) or delayed ones (e.g., infection and subclavian or internal jugular vein thrombosis).

PULMONARY ARTERY (SWAN-GANZ) CATHETERS

The gold standard for invasive hemodynamic monitoring is the pulmonary artery (PA) catheter (commonly called Swan-Ganz catheter). This flow-directed, balloon-tipped catheter traverses the right heart and enters a PA. It allows measurement of right atrial and PA pressures, as well as pulmonary capillary wedge pressure (PCWP), which is an estimate of left ventricular end diastolic pressure. In addition, it can sample mixed venous blood from the PA and calculate cardiac output using the thermodilution technique (see Measured Parameters).

Indications

Indications for use of PA catheters in surgical patients are varied. In general, their use should be in patients in whom the measured and calculated parameters guide or determine patient management. The common indications to be considered are listed here.

- For pre-, intra-, and postoperative management of high-risk patients (e.g., those with significant cardiac dysfunction or extensive operation)
- For hemodynamically unstable patients requiring inotropic or vasopressor support
- For determination of hydrational status in patients with equivocal findings
- For patients with adult respiratory distress syndrome requiring high positive end-expiratory pressure (PEEP) therapy

Device

Standard catheters are 110 cm long and have three or four lumens or ports along their distal 30 cm (Fig. 28–1). When properly placed, one lumen is in the right atrium, a second optional lumen is in the right ventricle, a third lumen is at the distal tip of the catheter in the PA, and the fourth lumen allows inflation and deflation of the balloon at the tip.

The temperature-sensitive thermistor required for cardiac output determinations is located just proximal to the catheter tip. Specialized catheters are available with cardiac pacing wires and pulse oximetry capabilities.

Insertion

The following steps are guidelines for insertion of a PA catheter:

1. Immediately before insertion, a sheath (Cordis) introducer is placed into the internal jugular or subclavian vein using standard Seldinger technique. This introducer allows placement of the PA catheter through its center in addition to providing additional IV access.
2. Under strict sterile conditions, all catheter ports are flushed and tested. The catheter is inserted to 15 cm (superior vena cava or right atrium), and a CVP or right atrial pressure tracing should be visible on the monitor (Fig. 28–2).

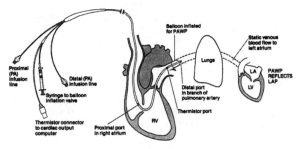

Figure 28–1. Lumens and proper position of a pulmonary artery catheter. (From Kersten LD [ed]. Comprehensive Respiratory Nursing: A Decision-Making Approach. WB Saunders, 1989, p 758, with permission.) PAWP = pulmonary artery wedge pressure; LAP = left atrial pressure; PAWP is equivalent to PCWP; LAP is equivalent to LVEDP = left ventricular end diastolic pressure.

3. The balloon of the catheter is inflated with 1.5 mL of air from its premeasured syringe. As the catheter is advanced (only with the balloon inflated), the flow of blood carries it into the right ventricle and then into the PA. (Lidocaine should be immediately available because ventricular arrhythmias induced by the catheter hitting the ventricular wall may occur.) As always, these catheter positions are confirmed by the appearance of characteristic pressure tracings (see Fig. 28–2).

4. The catheter is advanced farther into the PA until a "wedged" waveform is seen, indicating that the balloon is occluding a PA branch and the pressure sensed by its tip is coming from the left heart.

5. The balloon is deflated to ensure return of a PA tracing. The catheter is now ready for use.

A chest x-ray is obtained to rule out pneumothorax from the central venous puncture and to confirm proper catheter position.

Measured Parameters

The following parameters, with their normal ranges listed in parentheses, are measured by a PA catheter.

CVP (2 to 8 mm Hg). CVP is measured from the proximal or right atrial port. It provides an index of right-sided preload and is required for calculation of systemic vascular resistance (SVR).

PA pressures, systolic (20 to 30 mm Hg), diastolic (5 to 15 mm Hg) and mean PA pressures (9 to 16 mm Hg). These pressures are measured from the distal or PA

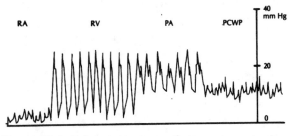

Figure 28–2. Pulmonary artery catheter pressure tracings. (From Shuck JM, Nearman HS. Technical skills in patient care. In Davis JH [ed]. Clinical Surgery. CV Mosby, 1987, p 711, with permission.)

port with the balloon deflated. The parameters provide a measure of pulmonary and left heart function. Mean PA pressure is required for calculation of pulmonary vascular resistance.

PCWP (2 to 12 mm Hg). Pulmonary capillary wedge pressure, or "wedge," is measured from the distal or PA port when the balloon is inflated. It is the best estimate of left ventricular end diastolic pressure (LVEDP), which is an assessment of left-sided preload.

CO (4 to 6 L/min). Cardiac output is determined by injecting a solution of known volume and temperature into the PA catheter's proximal port and measuring the change in temperature at the distal port by use of the catheter's thermistor. This is called the **thermodilution technique,** and the CO is determined electronically. CO provides a measure of cardiac function that is useful in the management of many clinical situations, particularly in hemodynamically unstable patients.

SvO$_2$ (65% to 75%). Mixed venous oxygen saturation is measured in a sample of blood obtained from the PA catheter's distal port. It is therefore the oxygen saturation of blood in its most desaturated state and provides an index of the body's oxygen requirements. Generally, a low SvO$_2$ value indicates inadequacy of oxygen delivery or increased oxygen utilization needs. SvO$_2$ is used to calculate the oxygen content of venous blood, which in turn is required for calculation of oxygen extraction ratio and intrapulmonary shunt.

Complications

In general, PA catheters are safe, but be aware of potential complications:

- Arrhythmias: premature ventricular contractions (PVCs), ventricular tachycardia, and fibrillation
- Catheter sepsis
- Pulmonary infarction
- Pulmonary artery rupture
- Catheter knotting

The bedside transducers of these catheters must be properly zeroed to a reference level on the patient (left atrium usually at midaxillary line). Thus, changes in the bed or patient's position may alter readings from any intravascular monitoring catheter.

29
CHAPTER

Running a "Code"

One of the most frustrating and bewildering experiences a medical student confronts is participating in a code or cardiac arrest. There is a flurry of activity that often seems disorganized, and it is difficult for the student to understand what is going on. This is compounded by the fact that the student is often assigned such tasks as performing cardiac compressions and obtaining an arterial blood gas. Although essential, these tasks tend to make it difficult to focus on the bigger picture of the conduct of the code.

The goal of this chapter is to present an outline of what causes most codes in a hospital setting and what should happen during these codes (e.g., Advanced Cardiac Life Support [ACLS] algorithms) based on several common clinical scenarios.

ETIOLOGY OF ARRESTS

The etiology of codes or arrests is manifold. Arrests can be divided into primary cardiac arrests and respiratory arrests. Some overlap exists in these classifications because if the heart develops a potentially fatal arrhythmia, breathing eventually stops. Conversely, ventilation that is impaired enough to cause severe hypoxemia or hypercarbia eventually leads to cardiac arrest.

Causes of cardiac arrest:

• Intrinsic cardiac disease (ischemia, arrhythmias)

- Hypoxemia
- Mechanical (tension pneumothorax, cardiac tamponade)
- Electrolyte disturbances (hypokalemia, hyperkalemia, hypomagnesemia)

Causes of respiratory arrest:

- Arrhythmias (bradycardia, asystole, pulseless electrical activity)
- Aspiration
- Tension pneumothorax
- Endotracheal tube obstruction (mucus plug, kinking)
- Ventilator malfunction

THE PRIMARY SURVEY

The first priority on arrival at the scene of a code is to determine whether the patient has indeed "coded" or is unresponsive. Determine this by rapidly asking the patient to respond verbally and by gently shaking the patient. If the patient does not respond, or gives a less than normal response, the next priority is to assess the patient's ABCDs. **PEARL: All codes begin with the primary ABCDs: airway, breathing, circulation, defibrillation.**

Airway—Open the airway. This includes use of the head tilt–chin lift maneuver (not in trauma patients) or jaw-thrust maneuver.

Breathing—Provide positive-pressure ventilation. The patient must either be breathing on his or her own or must be provided assistance breathing. At this stage, assistance may be in the form of a face-bag apparatus to "bag" the patient (most common) or mouth-to-face mask apparatus (less common). Intubation, if needed, occurs after defibrillation, below.

Circulation—Check for pulse and give chest compressions, if pulse is not present. An assessment of vital signs is made to determine the patient's pulse. The pulse should initially be sought at the neck (carotids), or the femoral arteries as a second choice. If a pulse is not felt, cardiopulmonary resuscitation (CPR) with closed-chest compressions is begun.

Defibrillation—The patient should be hooked up to the ECG leads of the crash cart to monitor cardiac electrical activity. At this point, if the rhythm is ventricular fibrillation (V-fib) or pulseless ventricular tachycardia (V-tach), up to three consecutive shocks (defibrillations at 200, 300, and 360 joules) should be delivered to restore a normal rhythm and pulse. The goal here is to look for and shock these reversible rhythms as quickly as possible.

THE SECONDARY SURVEY

The secondary survey is a more deliberate and detailed set of ABCs.

Airway

- Establish advanced airway control.
- Perform endotracheal intubation.

Breathing

- Assess adequacy of ventilation via endotracheal tube.
- Provide positive-pressure ventilation.

Circulation

- Obtain IV access to administer fluids and medications.
- Continue CPR.
- Provide rhythm-appropriate cardiovascular pharmacology.

Differential diagnosis

- Identify possible causes of arrest.
- Provide therapy, as clinically indicated, for reversible causes.

ACLS ALGORITHMS

Continued care of the patient is based on the patient's cardiac rhythm. There are five basic Advanced Cardiac Life Support (ACLS) algorithms, which dictate subsequent care during the code. Begin to be familiar with these complex algorithms. By the time you are an intern, you should have them memorized or keep them on a card in your pocket. The basic algorithms are for the following:

- Ventricular fibrillation/pulseless ventricular tachycardia
- Pulseless electrical activity (PEA; formerly termed electromechanical dissociation)
- Asystole
- Bradycardia
- Tachycardia

4
PART

Thoracic Surgery

30
CHAPTER

Chest Wall, Pleura, and Mediastinum

CHEST WALL TUMORS

Chest wall tumors can be classified by histologic type, by benign or malignant status (Tables 30–1 and 30–2), or by whether they are primary or metastatic from other sites. **PEARL: Most metastatic neoplasms to the chest wall are either carcinomas or sarcomas.** Neoplasms arising in the lung, breast, and pleura can become locally invasive to the chest wall. Most primary chest wall tumors are of cartilaginous or bony origin and are classified as sarcomas, and most chest wall tumors are malignant.

Workup includes a careful history, physical examination, and chest x-ray. MRI (magnetic resonance imaging) or CT (computed tomography) scan can be obtained to determine the anatomic extent of the lesion. Excisional biopsy is indicated for small tumors. Otherwise an incisional biopsy should be done within the future field of planned resection. Treatment options generally include wide excision.

PNEUMOTHORAX

A pneumothorax is defined as air in the pleural space. This is **collapsed lung** to the layperson. A pneumothorax may result in significant respiratory embarrassment

Table 30–1. BENIGN TUMORS OF THE CHEST WALL

Type	Typical Symptoms	Age of Onset	Location	X-ray Findings	Treatment
Osteochondromas	None	Childhood	Rib metaphysis	Rim of calcification or "stippling," "ground glass," cortical thinning	Resect to prevent malignant degeneration
Fibrous dysplasia	Nontender	Early adulthood	Posterior lateral	Nonspecific	Wide excision
Desmoid	Nontender mass	Variable	50% shoulder/chest		Wide excision ± postop radiation therapy
Chondromas	Nontender mass	Variable	Anterior	Expansile with cortical thinning	Resect with wide margins (may look like low-grade sarcoma)

Table 30–2. MALIGNANT TUMORS OF THE CHEST WALL

Type	Typical Symptoms	Age	Location	X-ray Findings	Therapy	Prognosis
Chondrosarcomas	Painful slow-growing mass	Adult	Anterior	From medullary portion of bone	Excision	Survival 90–100%
Fibrosarcomas	Variable	Adult	Frequently invade muscle and bone	Indistinct margins	Excision, chemotherapy, and radiation therapy	5-yr survival 50%
Ewing's sarcoma	Painful	Adolescent, female>male	Variable	"Onion skin"	Chemotherapy and radiation therapy; surgery for biopsy and residual disease	5-yr survival 50%
Osteogenic sarcoma	Painful/rapid growth	Adult	Lung nodules frequently associated	"Sunburst"	Chemotherapy, then excision	5-yr survival 20%
Plasmacytomas	Pain without a mass (many develop multiple myeloma)	Adult	Variable	Osteolytic "punched out"	Chemotherapy and radiation therapy	

Continued on the following page

Table 30–2. MALIGNANT TUMORS OF THE CHEST WALL (continued)

Type	Typical Symptoms	Age	Location	X-ray Findings	Therapy	Prognosis
Malignant fibrous histiocytoma	Slow growth	Older adults	Variable	Nonspecific	Excision followed by radiation therapy	
Rhabdomyosarcoma	Painless mass	Children and young adult	Skeletal muscle	Soft tissue tumor	Chemotherapy and radiation therapy	

and can present an emergency situation. Pneumothoraces are commonly **spontaneous** or **traumatic:**

- Spontaneous pneumothorax occurs in patients with chronic obstructive pulmonary disease (COPD) or in thin, young male patients with asthenic habitus. Catamenial pneumothoraces occur in concert with the onset of menstruation in young women.
- Traumatic pneumothorax can occur after penetrating trauma or attempts at central venous catheter insertion.

PEARL: The percentage of pneumothorax is calculated by averaging the distance in centimeters from lung to chest wall apically, laterally, and basally. This number is then converted to a percentage with a nomogram or can be roughly estimated by multiplying by 10.

Treatment Considerations

The specific treatment of a pneumothorax is context-dependent. The following are treatment considerations for pneumothorax.

- For a first-time pneumothorax, treatment is influenced by the presence or absence of symptoms, the size of the pneumothorax, and the condition of the underlying lung. Pneumothoraces of 25% or less can be observed in otherwise healthy patients with minimal symptoms.
- Chest tube drainage is indicated in patients with more than 25% collapse on chest x-ray, tension pneumothorax, increasing symptoms, increasing size of the pneumothorax on successive films, or significant disease in the contralateral lung.
- Effusions associated with pneumothoraces usually represent a complicated hemothorax and require thoracostomy drainage.
- Approximately 4% of patients will *not* have adequate expansion of the affected lung after thoracostomy tube placement. In most, however, the lung will expand and the air leak will seal within 24 to 48 hours. For persistent air leak, the patient may require thoracoscopic or open bleb stapling or pleurodesis.

- Operation for pneumothorax involves oversewing or stapling the affected area with or without pleurectomy. A mechanical or chemical pleurodesis can also be accomplished with tetracycline, mechanical irritation, or talc powder. Talc pleurodesis is rarely indicated for benign disease.

Recurrence

The risk of recurrence of pneumothorax is estimated at 20% after the first episode in patients who do not have COPD. After a second recurrence, the risk of recurrence rises to 60% to 80%. Three quarters of recurrent pneumothoraces occur on the same side within the first two years after the initial event.

Risk factors for recurrence of pneumothorax include:

- More than one previous episode
- COPD
- An air leak that persisted for more than 48 hours
- Tube drainage for less than 24 hours
- Complicated pneumothorax
- Systemic infection associated with the first event

In COPD patients, the air leaks are typically multicentric, and morbidity and mortality are significantly increased. The risk of recurrence after the first pneumothorax is 50% in patients with COPD, compared with 20% in the general population.

Early intervention with thoracoscopy may limit the risk of recurrence and diminish the rate of recurrence. This could offer overall cost savings in patients with pneumothoraces.

PLEURAL EFFUSION AND EMPYEMA

In evaluating patients with empyemas or pleural effusions, it is important to be able to make the distinction between an exudate and a transudate (Table 30–3). Exudates suggest the need for chest tube drainage, whereas a transudate may respond to medical therapy.

Empyemas, or septic effusions, should be considered as a separate entity from simple effusions. Empyemas develop in the following three stages:

Table 30–3. CHARACTERISTICS OF PLEURAL EFFUSIONS

	Exudate	Transudate
pH	<7.2	>7.2
Glucose (ng/dL)	<60	>60
Protein (ng/dL)	>3	
Protein fluid/serum	>0.5	
Lactic dehydro-genase (LDH)	>200	
LDH fluid/serum	>0.0	
Color	Bloody turbid yellow with pancre-atitis or esophageal perforation	Clear, straw-colored
Amylase	Increased	Serum normal or less

- Acute or exudative stage. The fluid is generally free-flowing, and thoracentesis and antibiotics are the treatment of choice.
- Fibropurulent stage. Loculated collections are seen with the fibropurulent stage and require surgical drainage.
- Final stage. If the lung is scarred down and fails to expand, the patient may be in the final stage of empyema development. A thoracotomy with drainage of the abscess cavity, debridement of fibrous peel, and placement of large thoracostomy tubes is indicated.

If an extensive pleural peel is noted, **decortication** (extensive debridement of pleural peel) should be considered. An option for patients with underlying COPD is pleural instillation of urokinase in an attempt to loosen the peel.

MALIGNANT PLEURAL EFFUSIONS

Malignant pleural effusions are defined as the presence of malignant cells in pleural fluid. Malignant effusions develop as a result of compromised lymphatic drainage of the pleura. As large volumes of fluid are generated that cannot be absorbed at the level of the mediastinal nodes, the fluid accumulates in the pleural space.

Signs and Symptoms

The following are findings in patients with malignant pleural effusions:

- Most patients present with shortness of breath, which may be progressive.
- The fluid that is aspirated may be bloody or serous in appearance with more than 100,000 red cells per square milliliter.
- The protein level is generally slightly elevated with somewhat depressed glucose concentration.
- Fluid cytology remains the cornerstone of diagnosis. However, pleural biopsy (percutaneous, thoracoscopic, or open) may be required to confirm the diagnosis.

Treatment

PEARL: Treatment for malignant effusions is palliative (tube drainage), because most affected patients are not candidates for curative resection. The exception is certain patients with Hodgkin's disease and non-Hodgkin's lymphoma, who may respond well to chemotherapy and radiation therapy.

If drainage is persistent, sclerotherapy with tetracycline, bleomycin, heat-inactivated BCG, or talc may be indicated. These agents are instilled into the pleural space to accomplish chemical pleurodesis. Tetracycline is effective in 70% to 80% of patients long-term, and talc poudrage offers a success rate of approximately 90% in patients with malignant effusions.

Pleural-peritoneal one-way pumps may be implanted subcutaneously. These pumps are activated by a patient's device when symptoms arise.

MEDIASTINAL MASSES

Mediastinal masses are classically categorized according to their anatomic location:

- **Anterior mediastinum.** PEARL: Anterior mediastinal masses begin with "T" and include thymomas, teratomas, parathyroid and thyroid gland, and testicular tumors (seminomatous or germ cell).
- **Middle mediastinum.** These masses include cysts that can be bronchogenic or pericardial and most commonly represent lymphadenopathy secondary to granulomatous disease, lymphoproliferative disease, or sarcoidosis.
- **Posterior mediastinum.** These mediastinal masses include mesotheliomas, esophageal duplication cysts, and, most typically, neurogenic tumors.

Children tend to have a preponderance of neurogenic tumors and less commonly present with lymphomas or mediastinal cysts. Approximately 30% of patients afflicted with myasthenia gravis have an associated thymoma.

Most mediastinal masses are asymptomatic and are found on chest x-ray or CT scan during an evaluation for an unrelated illness. The chest x-ray should be thoroughly reviewed and a chest CT scan obtained.

A tissue diagnosis is usually required, often using a percutaneous needle biopsy. This may be possible with posterior mediastinal masses, but anterior and middle mediastinal masses may require mediastinoscopy. Mediastinoscopy does not access the left aspect of the middle mediastinum well, and a Chamberlain procedure (limited thoracotomy) may be required.

Serum markers should be measured. Elevated catecholamine levels may reflect the presence of pheochromocytoma or neuroblastoma and α-fetoprotein (AFP), human chorionic gonadotropin (HCG), or carcinoembryonic antigen (CEA) may be elevated in patients with germ cell tumors. Iodine-131 (^{131}I) scanning and sestamibi scanning can be useful in investigating for substernal thyroid and parathyroid tissue.

Treatment Options

PEARL: In general, mediastinal tumors require excision. Unless highly suspicious for lymphoma or germ cell tumor, a preoperative tissue diagnosis is not required. The following are options for treating masses in the mediastinum:

- Symptomatic substernal goiters are resected. However, for substernal thyroids with no chemical evidence of a medullary carcinoma and no significant airway compression, medical treatment with suppressive doses of thyroxine may suffice.
- Lymphomas and granulomatous diseases require only biopsy for diagnosis and are subsequently treated medically.
- Seminomatous and nonseminomatous tumors require biopsy for diagnosis and an excision of the primary. Seminomas are treated with radiation therapy to nodal disease.
- Nonseminomatous tumors are treated with chemotherapy followed by excision of residual lymph node disease.
- Neurogenic tumors are best treated with wide surgical excision followed by postoperative radiation therapy and chemotherapy.
- Teratomas and thymomas are best treated with complete excision.

31

CHAPTER

Esophagus

ESOPHAGEAL ANATOMY

The esophagus has two muscular layers: an outer longitudinal layer and an inner circular layer. It is lined by squamous epithelium approximately down to the gastroesophageal junction. The upper esophageal sphincter (UES) or cricopharyngeus muscle is at the level of the sixth cervical vertebra (C6). The lower esophageal sphincter (LES) is a high-pressure zone that is poorly defined anatomically and is found at the level of the tenth thoracic vertebra (T10).

During endoscopy, the UES is found 15 cm from the incisors, and the LES is found 40 cm from the incisors. These anatomic relationships are very consistent in the adult population.

ESOPHAGEAL DYSMOTILITY

Evaluation of patients with dysphagia and odynophagia typically begins with a barium swallow, followed by esophagoscopy. A barium swallow is easily obtained and provides a roadmap for subsequent potential endoscopy and surgery. It is only 50% sensitive for the detection of gastroesophageal reflux disease (GERD). Rigid esophagoscopy is typically used for biopsy and stricture dilation, but initial diagnostic studies are more commonly performed with flexible endoscopy. Esophageal function tests may also be required.

Manometry is used to examine patterns of peristalsis and to look for normal LES relaxation after swallowing. The more sensitive measure of GERD is 24-hour pH probe monitoring. Patients keep a diary of diet and activity, which will be compared with pH recordings.

Functional Disorders

Functional diseases of the esophagus lack an anatomic abnormality and involve abnormal patterns of muscular contraction associated with swallowing (Table 31–1).

Diverticula

Pulsion diverticula are distributed in the cervical esophagus (Zenker's diverticulum) or lower esophagus (epiphrenic diverticulum). Treatment consists of diverticulectomy in combination with esophageal myotomy distal and proximal to the diverticulum.

Scleroderma

Scleroderma is characterized by loss of effective peristalsis and competency of the LES. With scleroderma, GERD can become severe.

Achalasia

Achalasia is dilatation of the esophagus caused by a failure of relaxation of the LES. As effective peristalsis is lost, the entire esophagus becomes dilated. Chest x-rays may demonstrate the so-called megaesophagus with "bird beak" tapering of the obstructed distal esophagus. Ten percent of affected patients will develop malignant changes.

Treatment of achalasia is initially medical with pneumatic dilation of the LES (effective in two-thirds of patients). With relief of obstruction of the LES, a pattern of normal peristalsis may return to the body of the esophagus. With failure of medical therapy including

TABLE 31–1. FUNCTIONAL DISORDERS AND DIVERTICULA OF THE ESOPHAGUS

Disorder	Mechanism/Finding	Treatment
Neurogenic dysphagia or cricopharyngeal dysfunction	UES fails to relax with swallowing; "posterior bar" on barium swallow.	Dilation or cervical myotomy
Diffuse esophageal spasm	Secondary to gastroesophageal reflux irritation or may be idiopathic; "corkscrew" on barium swallow.	Calcium channel blockers, nitrates, psychotherapy
Zenker's diverticulum	High-pressure zone secondary to failure of UES relaxation. Leftward posterior pouch on barium swallow; 25% of barium swallows are normal.	Myotomy proximal and distal to diverticulum usually in combination with diverticulectomy
Epiphrenic diverticulum	LES fails to relax, develop pulsion diverticulum within 10 cm of diaphragm on barium swallow.	Myotomy and diverticulectomy if > 3 cm, if symptomatic, or if operating on esophagus for another reason
Fraction diverticulum	Wide-mouthed pouch in mid-esophagus due to granulomatous disease.	Diagnosis and treatment of underlying condition; repair of any fistulas
Achalasia	Failure of LES relaxation and loss of peristalsis.	See text (dilation myotomy; possible esophagogectomy if unsalvageable)
Scleroderma	Loss of peristalsis and LES tone leads to severe reflux.	Medical (see text)
Shatzki's ring	Implies presence of type I hernia; symptomatic if <12 mm diameter.	Dilation ± antireflux procedure

VES = upper esophageal sphincter
LES = lower esophageal sphincter

pneumatic dilation, operative esophageal myotomy is indicated and is effective in 90% of patients. With esophageal myotomy the gastroesophageal sphincter is often rendered incompetent, and an antireflux operation is done at the time of operation. This disease is progressive, and advanced cases may require esophagectomy and recontruction.

Hiatus Hernia

Hiatus hernia and GERD are not synonymous. Either condition may occur without the other.There are classically four types of hiatus hernia:

- Type 1 is a sliding hiatal hernia (Fig. 31–1). **PEARL: Sliding hiatal hernia is commonly associated with GERD and is the most common type of hiatal hernia.**
- Type 2 is a paraesophageal hernia (Fig. 31–2).
- Type 3 is a combined hernia.
- Type 4 is a severe form of paraesophageal herniation with either the entire stomach or additional organs present within the thorax (Fig. 31–3).

Paraesophageal hernias are not commonly associated with reflux disease but place the patient at risk for incarceration, obstruction, chronic bleeding, and perforation. Therefore, all paraesophageal hernias should be repaired if the patient is fit for operation.

Symptoms and Complications

Symptoms of GERD include heartburn and effortless regurgitation, both of which may be made worse by assuming the supine position.

Complications of GERD include the following:

- Aspiration
- Bleeding secondary to esophagitis
- Dysphagia, which maybe secondary to spasm stricture
- The development of Barrett's esophagus.

PEARL: Barrett's esophagus is defined by the presence of columnar epithelium at least 3 cm above the gastroesophageal junction. Malignant degeneration is thought

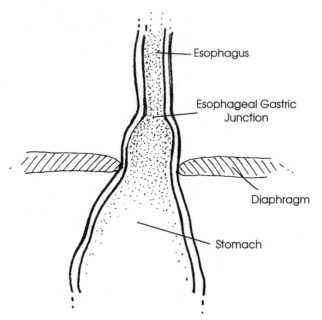

Figure 31-1. Sliding hiatus hernia. Note that the esophageal gastric junction is above the diaphragm.

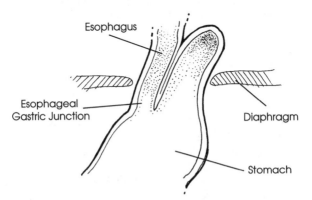

Figure 31-2. Paraesophageal hernia. Note that the esophageal gastric junction is in its normal position.

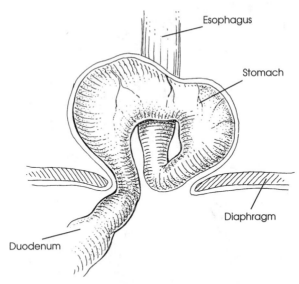

Esophagus

Stomach

Diaphragm

Duodenum

Figure 31–3. Paraesophageal hernia with herniation of the entire stomach to the thorax.

to occur in approximately 5% to 15% of patients, depending on the degree of dysplasia seen on biopsy. With severe dysplasia, this risk equals 25%. The diagnostic evaluation of GERD should always include esophagoscopy to evaluate the severity of esophagitis and the possibility of malignancy.

Treatment

Treatment of esophageal reflux is initially medical and is effective in 75% to 90% of patients. Treatment measures include the following:

- Weight loss
- Antacids
- Limitation of smoking and alcohol
- Histamine-(H_2-)blockers
- Prokinetic agents
- Elevation of the head of the bed

- Avoidance of tight clothing
- Limitation of oral intake several hours before bed-time

Surgery

The two most common surgical repairs for GERD are the Nissen and the Belsey repairs.

- The **Nissen repair** is a 360-degree wrap of the fundus of the stomach around the distal (intra-abdominal) esophagus. This creates a new high-pressure zone in the distal esophagus. The Nissen can be performed open or laparoscopically.
- The **Belsey repair** is a 240-degree anterior fundoplication. This is preferred to the Nissen when esophageal peristalsis is subnormal.

Indications for antireflux operation are:

- Paraesophageal hernias
- Type I hernias with:
  - Refractory symptoms
  - Ulcerative esophagitis
  - Complications of GERD (e.g., significant bleeding, recurrent stricture, repeated aspiration, malnutrition)

The presence of Barrett's esophagus is considered by some authors to be an indication for antireflux operation.

CONTROVERSY: Current belief is that patients with Barrett's metaplasia should undergo antireflux operation only if they meet the general indications described for GERD.

Patients with Barrett's and severe dysplasia should be considered for esophagectomy, because microscopic foci of invasive carcinoma are often found.

About 90% of esophageal reflux strictures can be dilated to at least a 46F size (about 15 mm) to allow comfortable swallowing. Two questions must first be answered:

- Is the stricture benign or malignant (determined with esophagoscopy and biopsy)?
- Is the stricture dilatable?

Esophagectomy may be indicated for GERD in the following situations:

- Severe dysplasia in an area of Barrett's metaplasia
- Perforation in the face of a dilated proximal esophagus with poor peristalsis
- An undilatable stricture
- Malignancy within a Barrett's esophagus

In the latter instances, the desired surgical approach is a transhiatal esophagectomy.

BENIGN ESOPHAGEAL LESIONS

There are two types of benign esophageal tumors: epithelial (papillomas, polyps, adenomas, and cysts) and nonepithelial (myomas, vascular tumors, and other mesenchymal tumors). Rarely, ectopic thyroid, pancreatic, gastric, and submandibular gland tissue may be found in the esophagus.

PEARL: Leiomyoma is the most common benign tumor of the esophagus but is still relatively rare. These lesions are typically asymptomatic, round or oval, and well circumscribed. They have a smooth surface and are covered by normal mucosa. The diagnosis is made with endoscopy and barium swallow. Leiomyomas should be resected.

ESOPHAGEAL CANCER

Two histologic subtypes of esophageal cancer exist: squamous cell cancer and adenocarcinoma. Squamous cell cancer is the most prevalent histologic type worldwide, but in the United States adenocarcinoma is becoming more common than squamous.

Risk factors for the development of carcinoma include the following:

- Prior caustic injury
- Cervical esophageal webs
- Diverticula (Zenker's, possibly)
- Excessive smoking and alcohol consumption
- Certain nutritional deficiencies
- The presence of achalasia or Barrett's esophagus
- Tylosis palmaris et plantaris

Approximately 50% of patients who present with adenocarcinoma of the esophagus have Barrett's metaplasia in the remaining esophagus. **PEARL: Aggressive medical therapy for Barrett's metaplasia in the form of reflux medication and antacids does not protect against progressive dysplasia or the development of cancer. Similarly, antireflux surgery does not protect the patient with Barrett's esophagus against the progression of malignancy.**

Because the esophagus is an elastic, distensible tube, peristaltic movement of a food bolus is not impaired until a lesion is sizable. Thus, most patients with carcinoma of the esophagus present late with dysphagia. Patients should be evaluated with barium swallow and endoscopy. The latter is needed for a tissue diagnosis. A CT (computed tomography) scan should be performed to identify the extent of disease and to look for lymphadenopathy. Esophageal endoscopic ultrasound is useful in accessing the depth of invasion and nodal enlargement.

Treatment and Prognosis

Treatment for esophageal carcinoma continues to evolve but is most effective when a multimodality approach is used. Radiation therapy alone is associated with a cure rate of approximately 10%. Postoperative radiation therapy appears to diminish local recurrence rates but does not increase long-term survival. Many centers start with esophagectomy.

Multiagent chemotherapy combined with preoperative radiation therapy has shown to cause significant regression of gross disease at the time of surgery.

CONTROVERSY: If residual disease is not seen after preoperative chemotherapy and radiation therapy, esophagectomy is advised by many authorities, and enhanced survival is anticipated.

Chemotherapy in combination with radiation therapy followed by surgical excision of the esophagus may offer improved 5-year survival compared with surgery alone or surgery with postoperative radiation therapy. Esophagectomy is accomplished via right thoracotomy combined with an abdominal incision (Ivor-Lewis procedure) or via a transhiatal and cervical approach without thoracotomy. After surgical excision of the esophagus, reconstruction may be accomplished using the stomach, jejunum, left colon, or right colon. Conduits may be placed in the retrosternal route or, preferably, in the bed of the resected esophagus.

Patients who are not candidates for curative resection are considered for palliation.

CONTROVERSY: Some centers offer esophagectomy as effective palliation, whereas many consider the morbidity and mortality to be prohibitive.

Major goals of palliation are relief of dysphagia and restoration of lumen, allowing the patient to eat. Radiation offers effective palliation in more than 75% of patients. Phototherapy with porphyrin sensitization and laser debulking with or without endoluminal stenting offer attractive alternatives at selected centers.

The 5-year survival rate for carcinoma of the esophagus is less than 10%. This is because most patients present with late stages of the disease. **PEARL: Approximately two-thirds of patients with esophageal carcinoma are inoperable at the time of presentation because of advanced disease.**

32
CHAPTER

Lungs

Thoracic surgeons are most frequently consulted in cases that indicate lung neoplasm. The most common situation is that of a patient with a smoking history who has new-onset, blood-streaked sputum, weight loss, or an abnormal chest x-ray. Other situations that raise suspicion of lung neoplasm include the presence of postobstructive (tumor) pneumonia and frank hemoptysis.

This chapter focuses on pulmonary neoplasms. For information on pulmonary infections and pulmonary insufficiency, see Chapter 26.

LUNG NODULES

Diagnostic Procedures

In patients with pulmonary nodules, the following methods should be carried out:

- Inquire about any history of granulomatous disease, smoking. Any symptoms related to the chest or respiratory system are critical.
- Obtain any previous chest x-rays to evaluate whether the nodule has been present for any interval of time. Unless the pulmonary nodule can be identified as old granulomatous disease or scar by previous chest x-rays, a tissue diagnosis is required.

- Order a CT scan of the chest, if indicated, to further evaluate the nodule and detect any mediastinal adenopathy. This is important staging information, because patients with lung cancer and mediastinal adenopathy are not resectable for cure.
- Evaluate central (perihilar) masses with three consecutive specimens of sputum for cytology. A flexible bronchoscopy with brushings and washings should be planned.
- Peripheral lesions may be evaluated with percutaneous needle biopsy under CT guidance; however, this is typically necessary for patients who cannot tolerate an operation (so they may receive palliative treatment). Suspicious nodules in all other patients should be resected.
- Evaluate questionable lymph node involvement on CT scan with transbronchial biopsy or mediastinoscopy.

Left lower lobe pulmonary malignancy is associated with right-sided positive hilar nodes in approximately one-third of patients. Such nodal positivity precludes a curative resection. Thoracotomy ultimately may be required for diagnosis and determination of resectability when the results of less invasive tests are not definitive.

LUNG CANCER

Lung cancer is the most common cause of cancer-related deaths in both men and women. **PEARL: By far the most common risk factor for the development of lung cancer is cigarette smoking.** The three most common types of lung cancer are:

- Adenocarcinoma
- Squamous cell carcinoma
- Small-cell carcinoma.

Squamous cell and small-cell tumors tend to be central, whereas adenocarcinomas are more frequently located in the periphery of the lung (exceptions to this are not uncommon).

Requirements for Resection

Surgical resection requires anatomic resectability (e.g., no involvement of hilar vessels) and physiologic resectability (i.e., pulmonary reserve). **PEARL: Before surgery for pulmonary resection, patients should be evaluated for their ability to tolerate a pulmonary resection.** Arterial blood gas values, pulmonary function tests, and split-function V-Q scans may be required to complete the preoperative assessment. In patients with normal exercise tolerance, pulmonary function tests are rarely compromised to the extent that resection is precluded. However, if any limitation is noted in forced expiratory volume in 1 second (FEV_1) on pulmonary function testing, a V-Q scan should be obtained to determine a contribution of each lung to the predicted postoperative FEV_1. A predicted postoperative FEV_1 of at least 0.8 L is required to ensure that the patient will tolerate the resection.

Risks for Complications

Patients with the following are considered to be at increased risk for developing complications after surgery:

- Mandatory minute volume (MMV) less than 40% predicted
- FEV_1 less than 60% predicted
- Po_2 less than 60 or Pco_2 greater than 45 (room air)

Contraindications to Surgical Resection

Patients who are *not* candidates for anatomic resection (i.e., those whose FEV_1 is less than 60% of predicted) may still be candidates for wedge resection.

CONTROVERSY: Wedge resections are associated with a higher incidence of postoperative recurrence, and several recent studies suggest compromised long-term survival for patients who undergo subanatomic resection.

Table 32–1 contains a list of contraindications to resection.

Table 32–1. CONTRAINDICATIONS TO RESECTION FOR LUNG CANCER (NON–SMALL-CELL)

N3 lesions (contralateral nodes, scalene nodes, supraclavicular nodes)

T4 lesions (malignant effusions, invasion of mediastinal sarcomas)

M1 lesions (extrathoracic metastases)

Bulky N2 disease (controversial)

Selected T3 lesions (chest wall invasion with positive nodes)

Management

Surgical resection in appropriate patients should include a lobectomy or a pneumonectomy, depending on the extent of the tumor. A concurrent dissection or sampling of the hilar nodes on the affected side should also be done. Postoperative radiation therapy and possibly chemotherapy are indicated if positive nodes are found.

Treatment Considerations and Prognosis

The reader is advised to review a textbook for the TNM staging for lung cancer to understand operative indications and contraindications. The following are considerations regarding staging of tumors preparatory to surgery:

- T1 tumors are generally less than 3 cm.
- T2 tumors are larger than 3 cm.
- T3 tumors are within 2 cm of the carina or invade the chest wall, diaphragm, or surrounding pericardium.
- Invasion of the mediastinum implies the presence of a T4 tumor.
- N1 disease involves the ipsilateral hilar nodes.
- N2 disease involves the paratracheal and/or mediastinal nodes on the ipsilateral side.
- N3 disease implies positive nodes on the contralateral side or in the scalene position.

- M1 disease (as with other malignancies) implies the presence of distant metastases.

Palliative resections may be done for troublesome air leaks, bleeding, or postobstructive lung infections.

The 5-year survival rate for lung cancer in general is 10% to 15%. Localized cancer resected with curative intent has a 5-year survival rate of 65% for stage I (node-negative) lesions and 40% for stage II lesions.

Nonresectable lung cancers are frequently treated for palliation with chemotherapy and radiation therapy.

HEMOPTYSIS

Two important clinical problems for the thoracic surgeon are hemoptysis and lung abscess (see following section).

A patient who presents to the emergency room with massive hemoptysis must have diagnostic and therapeutic maneuvers performed *quickly*. Causes of hemoptysis include:

- Malignancy
- Pulmonary embolism (see Chapter 34)
- Bronchiectasis
- Tuberculosis
- Trauma
- Arteriovenous fistulas
- Lung abscesses

Typically, the vessels responsible for hemoptysis are bronchial arteries, not pulmonary arteries. **PEARL: Massive hemoptysis is defined as 500 to 800 mL of blood in a 24-hour period.**

Treatment

Patients with hemoptysis are not only at risk for exsanguination but are also at immediate risk of asphyxiation. Every attempt should be made to protect the uninvolved lung. As such, the patient should be turned with the presumed bleeding side down. Oxygen (100%) should be delivered, the patient should be fluid-resuscitated, and lab tests should be sent to prepare cross-matched blood. The patient should undergo rigid bronchoscopy in the operating room to more precisely identify the site of bleeding.

Bleeding from the left bronchus can be controlled with a large embolectomy catheter or Foley catheter passed through the rigid bronchoscope. Hemoptysis from the right bronchus is more difficult to control because the right upper lobe takeoff is not far from the carina. Therefore, it is easier to pass the endotracheal tube into the left mainstem bronchus to allow adequate oxygenation. Once the airway has been secured, the patient should be taken for angiography and the site of bleeding identified and potentially embolized.

If the latter maneuvers fail to control bleeding, the patient should undergo lobectomy or other pulmonary resection determined by endoscopic and angiographic identification of the site of bleeding.

LUNG ABSCESS

Lung abscesses most frequently develop in association with pneumonia, trauma, aspiration, or extension of local infection. **PEARL: Aspiration is the most common cause of lung abscess.** Fever, leukocytosis, and chronic disease states associated with aspiration favor lung abscess. The lack of these findings suggests cavitating carcinoma, particularly in a smoker.

Treatment

Sputum and blood cultures are obtained. If microbiologic results from these cultures are not satisfactory, additional cultures may be obtained using a transtracheal or transthoracic aspiration or via bronchoscopic brushings. Lung abscesses are initially treated with antibiotics and postural drainage. Bronchoscopy should be performed to examine for obstructing lesions, residual foreign bodies, or malignancies. If an absess has spontaneously decompressed into the airway, bronchoscopy may be unnecessary. If required, a rigid bronchoscope with adequate suction capacity is best.

CONTROVERSY: *Therapeutic benefit from bronchoscopy in these cases has not been definitively established.*

If patients remain febrile for two weeks during treatment, then percutaneous drainage of the abscess should be considered. Similarly, if a cavity persists for more than two months, percutaneous drainage of the cavity with potential instillation of antibiotic-containing solution should be considered. For extremely refractory cases, a limited thoracotomy should be considered.

33
CHAPTER

Acquired Heart Disease

Adult cardiac surgery involves two main procedures: valve replacement and coronary artery revascularization.

AORTIC STENOSIS

Aortic stenosis is typically asymptomatic until the later stages of disease. The heart undergoes concentric hypertrophy initially and becomes vulnerable to ischemia. Later, it may dilate or pump ineffectively, leading to poor systemic perfusion. Consequently, symptoms may include angina, syncope, or fatigue and signs of failure. Sudden death secondary to ventricular arrhythmias may also occur.

Clinical Findings

On examination, a systolic ejection murmur and diminished upstroke on peripheral pulses are evident. Cardiac enlargement may not be evident clinically or radiographically until the later stages of disease.

On catheterization left ventricular (LV) pressures exceed aortic pressures. However, this pressure gradient may diminish and left ventricular end–diastolic pressure (LVEDP) will rise, as will pulmonary capillary wedge pressure (PCWP).

Indications for Surgery

Indications for surgery for aortic stenosis include the following:

- The development of symptoms
- Evidence of ventricular decompensation
- Resting systolic gradient of 50 mm Hg or greater (**Caution:** This may drop as LV function decreases)

Valve-preserving operations are justified in young patients, but in most adults the valve should be replaced. Prosthetic valves are durable but require long-term anticoagulation. Tissue valves do not require anticoagulation but must be replaced in approximately 10 years.

CONTROVERSY: Systemic embolization is a risk with either valve (2% to 5% risk/patient-year).

AORTIC INSUFFICIENCY

The presentation of a patient with aortic insufficiency depends on the chronicity of the lesion. Sudden onset results in severe congestive heart failure (CHF), whereas slow onset allows the heart to handle the gradual increase in volume load and is reasonably well tolerated early on. Diastolic blood pressure drops, and as a result coronary perfusion may decrease. Later as the LV decompensates, LVEDP may rise significantly.

LV dilatation is the initial compensatory response, and cardiac enlargement is evident clinically and radiographically. PCWP rises, and although pulses have a rapid upstroke, arterial tracings may lack or demonstrate a delayed dicrotic notch.

Surgery is indicated for aortic insufficiency in the presence of the following:

- The development of symptoms
- A first episode of CHF
- Evidence of progressive LV dysfunction or cardiac enlargement

In general, numbers from cardiac catheterization do not correlate well with the need for operation. Again, except in the pediatric population, valve replacement is generally indicated.

MITRAL STENOSIS

Rheumatic disease generally involves the mitral valve more than the aortic valve. The appearance of a scarred, stenotic mitral valve may occur decades after the acute disease. Patients may be asymptomatic for years with mild mitral stenosis.

A diastolic rumble is characteristic of left atrial (LA) enlargement. Pulmonary congestion may be evident, particularly if atrial fibrillation is present and LA emptying is compromised. Pulmonary arterial pressure and PCWP are elevated at rest and may rise simply with exercise. Cardioversion (electrical or chemical) is desirable in patients with atrial fibrillation (A-fib). Patients may be supported with diuresis, fluid restriction, and digitalis.

Surgical therapy for mitral stenosis may involve commissurotomy or complex mitral repair. Severely damaged valves may require replacement.

Most patients with atrial fibrillation preoperatively remain in this rhythm postoperatively. Anticoagulation and antiarrhythmic agents are generally indicated for life.

MITRAL INSUFFICIENCY

Symptoms generally develop late in the course of mitral insufficiency and mainly include signs of congestive failure, such as fatigue wheezing. Atrial fibrillation and an apical heave may also be present. The murmur of mitral insufficiency is an apical systolic one. Left heart enlargement and pulmonary congestion are evident radiographically, and measured LA pressures are elevated with a prominent V wave.

Rheumatic disease may be the cause of mitral insufficiency. Other possible causes include myxomatous disease, dilated cardiomyopathy, papillary muscle ischemic rupture, endocarditis, and progressive prolapse.

Treatment

Diuresis and digoxin allow for successful management of symptoms, but surgery is indicated for patients with progressive CHF, marked cardiomegaly, or diminishing LV function. Again, valvuloplasty is frequently successful, but replacement may be inevitable. Operative mortality for valve repair or replacement for mitral insufficiency is greater than for mitral stenosis.

ISCHEMIC HEART DISEASE

Myocardial ischemia results from an imbalance between myocardial oxygen demand and supply. Medical therapy generally has a greater effect on decreasing demand, whereas percutaneous transluminal coronary angioplasty (PTCA) and surgery aim to increase supply.

Ischemic myocardium contracts poorly, relaxes poorly, and conducts abnormally. As a result, ischemia can lead to systolic and diastolic dysfunction (with low cardiac output) and arrhythmias.

Treatment

Medical

The cornerstones of medical therapy for ischemic heart disease include β-blockade, calcium channel blockade, and nitrates. Control of hypertension and hypercholesterolemia, diabetic control, and the cessation of smoking are also critical.

Surgery

The following are indications for revascularization:

- Disabling angina refractory to medical therapy
- Postinfarction angina
- Silent ischemia
- Angina in patients undergoing valve surgery

All these indications are predicated on patients having significant coronary disease with reconstructable vessels and significant myocardium at risk.

Conduit for bypass generally includes saphenous vein, but internal mammary arterial pedicle grafts have better long-term patency. Radial artery free grafts and gastroepiploic pedicle grafts may have some long-term benefits in younger patients.

Patients who experience the greatest benefit from surgical therapy include those with diminished LV function, left main disease or its equivalent, proximal left anterior descending artery disease (with right coronary artery or circumflex disease), and patients with three-vessel disease. *Complete revascularization* is critically important in patients with compromised LV function.

Risk factors for operative morbidity and mortality include the following:

- Diabetes
- Obesity
- Age over 70 years
- Creatinine greater than 2.0
- Forced expiratory volume in 1 second (FEV_1) of less than 1.5 liters
- Female sex
- Diminished LV function
- Poorly reconstructable vessels

Vein graft patency at 10 years after CABG is approximately 50%, whereas 90% of internal mammary grafts are patent 10 years after operation. Benefits of surgery include relief of angina, increased survival, increase in exercise capacity, and decrease in medication intake in most CABG patients.

CONTROVERSY: PTCA is improving and is currently being compared with CABG in the treatment of multivessel disease. However, PTCA and surgery should be viewed as complementary and not competitive treatment options. So far, diabetics and patients with decreased LV function still appear to benefit more from surgery. PTCA patients required frequent repeat interventions.

Medical therapies and less invasive procedures such as catheter-balloon angioplasty are gaining popularity for the treatment of patients with severe coronary artery disease. Similarly, minimally invasive techniques are being developed to allow operative coronary artery bypass surgery without large chest incisions.

5
PART

Vascular Surgery

34
CHAPTER

Peripheral Vascular Disease

PATIENT EVALUATION

Most patients with peripheral vascular disease have significant comorbidities. Approximately 30% of patients have severe coronary artery disease, 5% to 10% have had previous strokes, and many are hypertensive, diabetic, or smokers. The history should focus on risk factors in addition to symptoms specific to vascular disease.

Risk factors for atherosclerosis include the following:

- Smoking
- Diabetes
- Hyperlipidemias
- Clotting abnormalities
- Hypertension

Claudication

Claudication is muscle pain that is secondary to muscle ischemia and occurs with exercise. The pain is characterized as a cramping or heavy feeling and is relieved by rest. The location of the symptoms is determined by the level of disease. For example, femoropopliteal disease can result in calf claudication.

Thigh or buttock claudication is associated with aorto-iliac disease. It is important to document the distance walked before onset of claudication. **Rest pain** represents more advanced ischemic disease and is typically located over the metatarsal heads. Rest pain is sharp or burning and is aggravated by elevation (e.g., when the patient is recumbent at night). Conversely, dangling the feet over the bed often relieves symptoms.

Aortoiliac disease also can cause impotence secondary to hypogastric insufficiency. **PEARL: LeRiche syndrome is impotence and buttock claudication secondary to severe stenosis or occlusion within the aortoiliac distribution.**

Physical Examination

Physical examination of a patient with peripheral vascular disease must include a *well-documented pulse exam:*

- Carotid, brachial, radial, femoral, popliteal, and pedal pulses should be palpated and diagrammed.
- The extremities should be inspected for trophic changes as well as evidence of pallor, rubor, muscle wasting, dermatitis, cellulitis, or ulceration.
- An **ankle-brachial index** is obtained by measuring blood pressure at pedal and brachial arteries (Table 34–1). This is accomplished with a blood pressure cuff and a hand-held Doppler device.
- Bruits should be sought not only over the carotid and femoral positions but also in the abdomen.
- The abdomen should be examined for pulsatile masses (hypogastrium-abdominal aortic aneurysm; pelvis-iliac aneurysm).
- Skin ulceration should be well described in terms of location, size, and character. Ischemic ulcers tend to be painful and located over the toes. Venous stasis ulcers can be mildly uncomfortable and are more typically located around the ankles. Diabetic neuropathic ulcers are typically insensate and located at the heels or plantar surface of the metatarsal heads.
- When evaluating for chronic venous insufficiency, note evidence of infection, swelling, and brawny, brown induration.

Table 34–1. RELATION OF
ANKLE-BRACHIAL INDEX TO SYMPTOMS

Ankle-Brachial Index	Symptoms
1–1.15	None (normal)
0.6–0.8	Claudication
0.3–0.5	Rest pain
<0.3	Tissue loss

PEARL: Angiography is not a screening tool in cases of chronic peripheral vascular disease. Instead, an angiogram is obtained only when a vascular reconstructive procedure is indicated. Then, the angiogram allows for planning of the bypass operation.

ACUTE ARTERIAL INSUFFICIENCY OF THE EXTREMITIES

Successful management of acute arterial insufficiency depends on early diagnosis and aggressive institution of therapy (Table 34–2).

History and Physical Examination

A thorough history may allow differentiation between **embolic** and **thrombotic** causes of insufficiency.

Table 34–2. DURATION OF SYMPTOMS
AND MORBIDITY OF ACUTE
ARTERIAL INSUFFICIENCY

Duration of Symptoms	Ischemic Morbidity
<8 hours	20%
8–24 hours	30%
Several days	>40%

Embolic events are more common with a prior diagnosis of cardiac disease, especially atrial fibrillation and recent myocardial infarction. These patients typically do not give a history of prior vascular complaints. The most common site for embolic occlusion is the superficial femoral artery.

PEARL: The timing of the event is usually precisely described by the patient in terms of its abrupt onset and profound symptoms, such as the five p's: pain, pallor, paralysis, paresthesia, and poikilothermia. A recent episode of hypotension, especially compounded by dehydration, favors in situ thrombosis rather than embolic occlusion. **PEARL: Most patients presenting with acute thrombosis have a history of prior peripheral vascular complaints.**

Physical examination should focus on identifying cardiac dysrhythmias, manifestation of the five p's, and evidence of the peripheral malperfusion (e.g., collapsed superficial veins and poor capillary refill). Basic laboratory tests are of little value early except when profound muscle necrosis may have occurred, resulting in significant elevation in creatine phosphokinase and lactate and the presence of hyperkalemia and myoglobinuria. Chest x-ray and electrocardiogram (ECG) are indicated.

Treatment

The patient with acute arterial insufficiency of the extremities should be heparinized during the diagnostic workup. If significant muscle ischemia is suspected, the patient should receive mannitol, crystalloid, and sodium bicarbonate ($NaHCO_3$) to prevent crystallization of myoglobin in the renal tubules and ensure a brisk urinary output. If an embolic event occurred, an embolectomy is performed under local or regional anesthesia. Otherwise, the patient should be taken for angiography.

Recently thrombosed grafts and patients without reconstructable disease may be treated with thrombolytic therapy. An angiogram is used to plan a peripheral bypass should thrombectomy fail.

CHRONIC OCCLUSIVE LOWER EXTREMITY DISEASE

Atherosclerotic disease most commonly affects the lower extremities. There are specific patterns of distribution of occlusive lesions, such as the following:

- Lesions within the superficial femoral artery are classically at Hunter's canal.
- Lesions of the profunda femoris artery are typically ostial in distribution.
- Iliac lesions tend to be most severe at bifurcations.
- The aorta is commonly affected at the aortic bifurcation.
- The popliteal artery is most commonly diseased at the trifurcation and its distal extent.

Symptoms may include claudication, rest pain in the foot, or tissue loss (ulceration or gangrene). They reflect the level and severity of disease (aorto-iliac: hip and thigh pain; femoral-popliteal: calf pain). The presence of symptoms usually indicates the existence of significant disease at more than one level. This is particularly true of tissue loss, which indicates the presence of multiple levels of disease.

Physical examination is notable for diminution of distal pulses and trophic changes.

Treatment

Treatment of claudication mainly includes the following:

- Cessation of smoking
- Strict management of diabetes
- Control of hypertension
- Exercise

In addition, attempts should be made to alter serum lipid profiles. An exercise regimen should begin with patients advised to walk or exercise until they experience claudication, then rest briefly. They should repeat the cycle several times daily.

Remember that claudication itself generally follows a benign course. Of patients with claudication (no rest pain, no tissue loss), roughly one-third improve over time, one-third stabilize, and one-third get worse. Only 3% to 5% go on to amputation. Conversely, patients with rest pain or tissue loss are in jeopardy of limb loss. Patients with isolated claudication are not candidates for surgical revascularization unless their symptoms are quite debilitating.

PEARL: Patients who present with rest pain, tissue loss, disabling claudication, or other evidence of a threatened limb should be considered for revascularization. Only then is arteriography indicated, because it serves as a road map for reconstruction and not a physiologic index of blood flow.

Surgical Reconstruction

Surgical reconstructive options for femoropopliteal disease are determined by the location of disease in relation to the knee:

- When disease is limited to the femoropopliteal system, above-the-knee bypass with autologous vein or polytetrafluoroethylene (PTFE) can be considered. Long-term patency rates are similar when either of these two materials are used in this position.
- When disease extends below the knee, autologous vein has superior patency rates.

Type of Graft. Most surgeons use reversed saphenous vein. However, there are advantages with in situ saphenous bypass grafting. With this technique, the saphenous vein is exposed but left in its bed. The side branches are ligated, and valves are disrupted to render them incompetent. There is a better size match between the vein graft and the inflow and recipient arteries. In addition, the vasa vasorum are not disrupted. This theoretically offers less fibrosis or intimal hyperplasia compared with reverse saphenous vein.

CONTROVERSY: Composite grafts (vein plus prosthetic) may offer improved long-term patency compared with distal prosthetic grafts alone.

The need for a composite graft occurs when no saphenous vein of adequate length is available for below-knee bypass.

Sympathectomy. Sympathectomy has been previously used as an adjunct to vascular reconstruction. Sympathectomy increases blood flow to cutaneous tissues, but muscular blood flow is not improved. Long-term limb salvage rates are not significantly improved. Healing of skin ulcerations may temporarily be aided.

Nonsurgical

Selected patients may be candidates for nonsurgical revascularization. Catheter-guided atherectomy with stent placement in the iliac position offers significant long-term benefit.

Extensive experience with angioplasty in the infrainguinal positions is lacking, and long-term patency rates in the femoropopliteal distribution are poor.

Aortoiliac disease may be treated with stenting when iliac lesions are well localized. With the typical diffuse pattern of aortoiliac disease, aortofemoral grafting is required. Aortobifemoral grafting carries a patency rate of 85% to 95% at five years.

When patients are not medically fit to tolerate a major vascular operation, extra-anatomic grafts such as axillobifemoral grafting and femorofemoral cross-over grafting may be indicated. However, keep the following in mind:

- Femorofemoral bypass grafting requires that flow to at least one femoral artery be well preserved to ensure adequate inflow into the cross-over graft. Long-term patency approaches 75%.
- Axillobifemoral grafts have diminished long-term patency rates (50 to 65%) and a higher incidence of infection. Long-term patency may be improved when runoff is to both femoral arteries rather than to a unilateral axillofemoral graft.

PERIPHERAL ARTERIAL ANEURYSMS

Patients who have peripheral arterial aneurysms or abdominal aortic aneurysms are at significant risk for harboring arterial aneurysms in other locations. For example, patients with popliteal aneurysms have a 50% incidence of bilateral disease, and 60% have abdominal aortic aneurysms. Patients with femoral aneurysms have up to a 90% chance of harboring another aneurysm, and 10 to 20% of patients with abdominal aortic aneurysms have associated peripheral aneurysms. Following are the different types of aneurysms:

Iliac aneurysms are relatively rare and are typically asymptomatic. Patients classically first present with rupture, not thrombosis, and ecchymosis around the anus and genitalia may be present after contained rupture. Treatment generally involves bypass grafting with aneurysm exclusion or ligation.

Femoral aneurysms tend to present with thrombosis, and treatment is aneurysmorrhaphy or bypass.

Popliteal aneurysms commonly thrombose. Because they are functionally closer to being end-arteries, there is an associated high rate of limb loss.

Subclavian aneurysms are rare and may be caused by trauma, thoracic outlet syndrome, or atherosclerosis. Patients may present with thrombosis or rupture.

Carotid aneurysms tend to present as pulsatile neck masses. Patients are otherwise usually asymptomatic. Treatment involves aneurysmorrhaphy or resection with graft replacement.

Splenic artery aneurysms tend to occur in women of child-bearing age, especially those who are multiparous. The risk of rupture increases as splenic blood flow increases during pregnancy. Patients with aneurysms greater than 2 to 3 cm, women of child-bearing age, pregnant women with diagnosed splenic artery aneurysms, and patients with evidence of rupture should undergo repair.

Pseudoaneurysms do not contain all the layers of arterial wall. Postoperative pseudoaneurysms tend to occur secondary to graft separation owing to suture line breakdown or progressive degeneration of native arterial wall at the site of a vascular anastomosis. Anatomically, there is a break in the arterial wall with a fibrous capsule becoming the lining of the aneurysm. Pseudoaneurysms generally require repair if symptomatic or progressively enlarging. Size criteria also exist for replacement of pseudoaneurysms in various locations (e.g., femoral aneurysm greater than 2 cm requires repair).

Mycotic aneurysms are infectious in origin and may be caused by septic embolization, penetrating trauma, or inadvertent arterial puncture during attempts at intravenous drug abuse. Patients typically present with fever, pulsatile masses, and areas of cellulitis. Broad-spectrum antibiotics active against *Staphylococcus* and *Pseudomonas* should be instituted before final results of wound and blood cultures. Therapy generally requires resection, debridement, and, depending on limb viability, an extra-anatomic bypass through a noncontaminated field (obturator bypass in the case of femoral mycotic aneurysm).

DEEP VENOUS THROMBOSIS AND PULMONARY EMBOLISM

During daily activity, leg muscles act as pumps, periodically compressing deep leg veins, thus preventing stasis of blood. Many operations are performed with spinal anesthesia, epidural anesthesia, or general anesthesia with pharmacologic paralysis. These situations eliminate the leg muscle pump and promote venous stasis and thrombosis. Therefore, DVT and pulmonary embolism are known complications of surgery.

Risk factors for the development of deep venous thrombosis (DVT) and subsequent pulmonary embolism include:

- Hypercoagulable states
- Age greater than 40 years
- Prior history of DVT
- Pregnancy
- Obesity
- Estrogen therapy
- Malignancy
- Cardiac disease
- Prolonged bedrest
- Abdominal or pelvic surgery
- Trauma

PEARL: Virchow's triad for thrombosis is stasis, hypercoagulable state, and intimal injury.

Prevention of DVT is preferable to having to treat for DVT. Preventive measures for DVT are instituted pre-operatively:

- Subcutaneous heparin (5000 units) is administered every 12 hours, beginning 12 hours before surgery, for the greatest beneficial effect.
- Intermittent pneumatic compression stockings are best applied before induction of general anesthesia. The beneficial effects are directly proportional to the amount of muscle encompassed by the compression stocking. They function at least in part by increasing fibrinolytic activity.

Diagnostic Findings

Patients with DVT have inconsistent physical findings. Fifty percent of patients presenting with symptoms consistent with DVT will *not* have a DVT, and 50% of patients with DVT are asymptomatic.

PEARL: Homans' sign for DVT has been described (pain in the calf on dorsiflexion of the foot), but this finding is unreliable and is present in only one-third of patients with DVT.

With complete iliofemoral thrombosis, the leg may become deeply cyanotic and swollen (phlegmasia cerulea dolens). When venous hypertension is progressive, arterial inflow is compromised, and the leg may become pale and blanched (phlegmasia alba dolens). Without prompt institution of therapy, significant risk of limb loss is associated with this clinical syndrome.

Imaging

Duplex Doppler ultrasound has become the cornerstone of DVT diagnosis. Impedance plethysmography is approximately 80% to 90% sensitive for diagnosing proximal femoral thrombosis, and labeled fibrinogen studies are approximately 90% sensitive for diagnosing lower leg DVT. **PEARL: Venography represents the gold standard for diagnosing DVT with a virtual 100% sensitivity and specificity.**

Although venography is more sensitive and specific, venous Doppler ultrasound is more commonly used because Doppler studies are quick and noninvasive.

Treatment

Therapy for DVT includes limb elevation and continuous IV heparin to maintain a partial thromboplastin time (PTT) of 2 to 2.25 times the control. Following is a general treatment regimen:

- Oral anticoagulation with warfarin is instituted 1 to 2 days after heparin therapy is begun.
- After the prothrombin time (**PT**) reaches 1.5 to 2 times normal, heparin therapy can be stopped.
- Heparin is generally given for 1 week to allow for maximal clot retraction and maturation.
- Warfarin is continued for 3 to 6 months.

CONTROVERSY: Whether or not popliteal DVTs require anticoagulation therapy is controversial. Most authors agree that isolated infrageniculate popliteal thrombosis does not require therapy unless it shows evidence of propagation.

Diagnosis and Treatment of Pulmonary Embolism

Fortunately, only a minority of patients with DVT develop **pulmonary embolism.** With pulmonary embolism, the venous blood clot breaks free and circulates through the right side of the heart until it lodges in the pulmonary arterial circulation. This interferes with pulmonary blood flow and promotes the release of inflammatory mediators from the lung.

Such patients may present with dyspnea and chest pain (commonly) and may have hemoptysis (a late sign consistent with pulmonary infarction) or a pleural friction rub. Patients with large or multiple pulmonary emboli can present with circulatory collapse.

Chest x-ray changes are unreliable in these patients. ECG findings are classically described as an $S_1Q_3T_3$ pattern, but more typically demonstrate a sinus tachycardia and subtle signs of right heart strain. Arterial blood gas analysis may demonstrate a hypocarbia with preservation of a normal oxygen tension (pO_2). Patients may become hypoxic as the disease progresses.

Filter Placement

A vena caval filter looks like a badminton shuttlecock, but it is metallic. It is placed in the inferior vena cava via the jugular or femoral vein using a catheter system. The filter traps floating clots, thus preventing pulmonary emboli. With time those clots will dissolve.

The following patients are candidates for filter placement:

- Patients who have recurrent pulmonary embolization while adequately anticoagulated or have a complication of anticoagulation (e.g., gastrointestinal bleeding) or patients who have a contraindication to anticoagulation.
- Patients with a history of DVT
- Patients with free-floating thrombus
- Patients with a history of recurrent pulmonary emboli
- Patients with chronic thromboembolic pulmonary hypertension.

Thrombolectomy or Embolectomy

Occasionally, patients have massive embolization with associated circulatory collapse. This is associated with a greater than 50% mortality rate. These patients may require a suction catheter thromboembolectomy or operative embolectomy while on cardiopulmonary bypass. Success with this procedure is critically dependent on early diagnosis and swift mobilization to the operating room.

35
CHAPTER

Aorta

ABDOMINAL AORTIC ANEURYSMS

Nearly all abdominal aortic aneurysms (AAAs) are of atherosclerotic origin and begin below the level of renal arteries. Familial patterns and genetic associations have been identified among patients with AAAs. The rationale behind surgical therapy is best understood when one outlines the *risk* of rupture as it relates to aneurysm size:

- **PEARL: Aneurysms more than 6 cm in diameter have a greater than 40% risk of rupture.**
- Aneurysms smaller than 4 cm rarely rupture.
- Aneurysms 4 to 6 cm have a 20% risk of rupture and an associated mortality rate of slightly more than 50%.

Most surgeons agree that aneurysms larger than 6 cm require surgical therapy, and aneurysms 4 to 6 cm in good-risk patients should be repaired. Patients with AAAs smaller than 4 cm should be observed for development of symptoms or for a significant increase in size (by ultrasound exams at 6-month intervals).

Signs and Symptoms

Most patients with AAAs are asymptomatic. However, they occasionally present with abdominal pain,

269

back pain, or testicular pain suggestive of aneurysmal distention, leaking, or frank rupture. Typically, the asymptomatic patient is identified during routine physical examination as having a pulsatile abdominal mass.

A CT scan or an abdominal ultrasound demonstrates the presence and size of the aneurysm. Lateral abdominal x-rays may demonstrate calcification of the aortic wall at the aneurysmal margins.

Patients presenting with a ruptured or leaking AAA may manifest the following common classic triad:

- Abdominal or back pain
- Hypotension
- Pulsatile abdominal mass

Less common:

- Flank pain
- Testicular pain

If the patient remains hemodynamically stable, a CT scan (especially a rapid spiral CT scan) may be helpful to confirm the diagnosis. In a hypotensive patient, the CT scan is deferred and the diagnosis is confirmed in the operating room. Attempts at resuscitation to normal blood pressure are also ill advised because they may increase wall stress and precipitate free rupture.

Treatment

At least six to eight units of packed cells and component coagulation factors should be made ready for the operating room. AAAs are repaired by replacement of the infrarenal aorta with a synthetic graft.

Postsurgical Complications

Complications after surgery (particularly emergency surgery) include acute renal failure, disseminated intravascular coagulation (DIC), lower extremity ischemia, and ischemic colitis. The occurrence of any of these complications raises the mortality rate.

RENOVASCULAR DISEASE

Patients with significant atherosclerotic disease or fibromuscular dysplasia of the renal arteries may present with hypertension secondary to activation of the renin-angiotensin system. The mechanism of hypertension in these cases is as follows:

Diminished renal blood flow leads to increased renin production in the affected kidney. Renin increases angiotensin production with resultant peripheral vasoconstriction. Renin also induces aldosterone production, resulting in volume retention. Both the vasoconstriction and volume retention contribute to hypertension.

Assessment

Patients with hypertension of suspected renovascular origin should be assessed for hemodynamically significant renal artery stenosis. Workup may include assessment of renal vein renin level. Renal artery stenosis can be determined by the following venous renin measurements:

$$\frac{\text{[Renin] Renal vein (affected)}}{\text{[Renin] Renal vein (opposite side)}} \quad >1.5 = \text{Significant lesion}$$

$$\frac{\text{[Renin] Renal vein} - \text{systemic [Renin]}}{\text{Systemic [Renin]}} \quad >0.5 = \text{Significant lesion}$$

Patients without significant lesions by renal vein–renin ratios should undergo a captopril stimulation test to determine the likelihood that they will respond to surgical intervention. Captopril inhibits the conversion of angiotensin I to angiotensin II. Improvement of hypertension with this test predicts a good response to treatment for renal artery stenosis. In patients with bilateral renal artery stenosis (volume-dependent hypertension), renal vein renin ratios may be unreliable. Ratios are more reliable with unilateral renal artery stenosis (renin-dependent hypertension).

Treatment

Options for the treatment of renovascular disease include percutaneous balloon angioplasty and surgery.

Angioplasty is particularly appropriate for young women afflicted with fibromuscular hyperplasia. For non-ostial atherosclerotic lesions of the renal arteries balloon dilation is also a viable option. In general, atherosclerotic disease is less amenable to balloon dilation.

In surgical cases, flow to the diseased renal artery may be restored with aortic endarterectomies or bypass grafts to the renal arteries from the aorta, hepatic artery, or splenic artery.

MESENTERIC VASCULAR DISEASE

Acute

Acute mesenteric vascular occlusion is a surgical emergency of the highest priority. To make the diagnosis, the surgeon must have a high index of suspicion and be willing to use angiography early in the diagnostic algorithm. Frequently, this diagnosis is difficult to make because physical findings may be limited.

Signs and Symptoms

PEARL: Classically, patients with acute mesenteric ischemia are referred to as having *pain out of proportion to physical findings.* Typically, patients note an abrupt onset of symptoms (particularly when the cause is embolic) and describe their abdominal discomfort as severe, constant, and progressive. A common cause of mesenteric ischemia is a **low-flow state** due to left ventricular failure. Placement of a pulmonary artery catheter with measurement of cardiac output helps secure this diagnosis.

Patients with **embolic disease** may be identified by a history of atrial fibrillation, digoxin intake, recent myocardial infarction, or dysrhythmias that predispose to the development of cardiac mural thrombus and subsequent embolization.

Patients with acute mesenteric **thrombosis** typically have prior complaints of atherosclerotic occlusive disease and have recently become dehydrated or have been in a state of low cardiac output. Digoxin intake is also common in this population.

Regardless of the cause of mesenteric ischemia, a timely diagnosis and prompt institution of therapy are critical.

Evaluation and Management

Physical examination may reveal little abdominal tenderness until full-thickness intestinal infarction has occurred. With persistent ischemia, there may be acidosis, elevation of creatine phosphokinase and lactate, leukocytosis, and hematochezia. Patients with evidence of infarction (peritonitis or septic shock) should be taken to the operating room after a brief period of resuscitation to replace volume and correct acidosis. No additional studies are required before exploration. Necrotic bowel should be resected and the status of the mesenteric vasculature assessed.

It is important to remember that it is the patients who have *not* developed full-thickness infarction who are most likely to be saved by urgent operation.

CONTROVERSY: In patients without clinical evidence of full-thickness necrosis, there are two accepted approaches: exploratory laparotomy or angiography.

If the latter is chosen, both the celiac axis and the superior mesenteric artery (SMA) should be imaged. Angiographically, vascular thrombosis is characterized by ostial occlusion of the SMA. Emboli tend to lodge more distally and spare the first few jejunal branches of the SMA. At operation, the first portion of jejunum may be spared in patients with embolic occlusion of the SMA.

Once the diagnosis of mesenteric occlusion is suspected, the patient should begin heparin therapy. After the angiogram has been completed, papaverine (a vasodilator) may be infused through the arterial catheter. Patients with a history consistent with embolic occlusion may be taken directly to the operating room for embolectomy. If the cause of ischemia is confirmed as embolic, the embolus is extracted.

Doppler examination of the mesentery or inspection of the bowel after fluorescein injection using a Wood's lamp allows for assessment of viability. **PEARL: If any question remains about bowel viability, the bowel should be left in situ and the patient returned to the operating room 24 hours later for a second-look operation.** This allows nonviable bowel to declare itself, and the maximum length of bowel can be preserved. Patients with mesenteric **thrombosis** should be taken to the operating room after angiography and undergo removal of any possible clot. These patients are likely to require a bypass graft as well, because flow typically remains inadequate. Reconstructions are preferably done with saphenous vein as an aortomesenteric or iliomesenteric bypass.

Patients may also present with acute vascular insufficiency after repair of AAAs. This is secondary to inadequate collateral flow after ligation of an inferior mesenteric artery (IMA) (rectosigmoid ischemia). The diagnosis is made with sigmoidoscopy. Treatment of these patients generally involves resection of the ischemic segment of colon.

Acute mesenteric vascular insufficiency may occur with no evidence of anatomic obstruction. **PEARL: So-called nonocclusive mesenteric ischemia may occur in patients who are in states of severe low cardiac output.** Typically, these patients either have cardiac failure, are profoundly hypovolemic, or are septic. The diagnosis is suggested by low cardiac output. The diagnosis may be supported by angiography, which may demonstrate diminutive-appearing arterial runoff secondary to induced spasm. This condition is treated nonoperatively with cardiac-enhancing pharmaceuticals (e.g., dobutamine) and sometimes with a papaverine drip via the angiography catheter.

Chronic

Chronic mesenteric vascular insufficiency or "intestinal angina" is characterized by abdominal pain after eating and abdominal bruits. The pain causes patients to develop a fear of food, resulting in marked weight loss. Occlusion of two of three abdominal visceral vessels (celiac, SMA, IMA) is required to cause symptoms.

Treatment consists of surgical revascularization. In contrast to acute mesenteric ischemia (an emergency), chronic mesenteric insufficiency is treated with elective surgery.

36
CHAPTER

Cerebrovascular Disease

BACKGROUND

Atherosclerosis of the aortic arch and carotid and vertebral arteries constitutes cerebrovascular disease and is associated with significant morbidity and mortality. Emboli from or thrombosis of any of these vessels can result in severely disabling or life-threatening dysfunction of the central nervous system. Knowledge of the natural history of these problems has helped in the development of effective medical and surgical treatments. Keep the following in mind when examining a patient with suspected cerebrovascular disease:

- The incidence of cerebrovascular disease increases with age.
- The risk factors are the same as those for atherosclerosis in general—smoking, hypertension, hyperlipidemia, and diabetes.
- Symptoms such as severe headache, dizziness, syncope, sudden partial blindness, and paralysis all may be due to cerebrovascular disease. A detailed history covering each symptom is important.
- Equally important are performance and documentation of a detailed neurologic examination.

Transient ischemic attacks (TIAs) secondary to cerebrovascular disease are episodic symptoms of unilateral weakness, paralysis, or monocular blindness (which generally last no longer than 24 hours). Patients with TIAs have a risk of stroke of at least 5% to 6% per year.

Amaurosis fugax (brief temporary blindness) involves ipsilateral carotid disease, whereas motor symptoms involve contralateral carotid disease. **PEARL: Amaurosis fugax occurs after microembolization to a retinal artery and manifests as transient monocular blindness.** Unilateral hand, facial, or leg weakness may also occur.

Many other patients may have less typical findings of carotid disease, such as dizziness or motor discoordination, abnormalities in speech and comprehension, and, rarely, temporal lobe–related symptoms.

Frank stroke is a deficit that has persisted for more than 24 hours.

A **stroke in evolution** implies that some degree of deficit has persisted while the full extent of neurologic symptoms continue to develop while the patient remains under observation.

Although hemorrhagic strokes are typically associated with hypertension, strokes associated with occlusive disease are either of hypoperfusion or embolic etiology.

The acute mortality rate after a stroke is 15%. Also, the risk of recurrent stroke is 25% to 40%, and the mortality rate after recurrent stroke is greater than 60%. This readily justifies endarterectomy in patients who have had a stroke with significant neurologic recovery or persistent symptoms.

EVALUATION

After a detailed history and neurologic examination, the following diagnostic methods may be implemented:

- **PEARL: Duplex Doppler imaging has evolved in its accuracy and precision such that many surgeons operate based on vascular ultrasound examination alone.**
- Four-vessel angiography was previously required to adequately assess the anatomy before surgery. It is still required after Doppler examination if any question exists regarding the anatomic extent of obstruction.

- Early experience with the use of magnetic resonance angiography suggests that it may be a valuable noninvasive diagnostic tool.
- Ophthalmoplethysmography and assessment of periorbital blood flow continue to be used by a minority of clinicians as surveillance tools to examine for progression of disease during follow-up.
- Intravenous digital subtraction angiography (IVDSA) is another alternative to traditional angiography. IVDSA limits the risks of embolization associated with intra-arterial injection, but the contrast load used continues to place patients at risk for acute tubular necrosis, dehydration, and contrast allergies.

When evaluating any patient for possible carotid endarterectomy, it is critical to rule out other causes of the presenting symptoms. Specifically, patients should be examined for more proximal vascular disease, cardiac disease, and neurologic disorders.

CAROTID ENDARTERECTOMY

While aspirin therapy reduces the risk of stroke in patients with atherosclerosis of the cerebrovascular system, carotid endarterectomy plus aspirin reduces the relative risk of stroke 65% more than aspirin therapy alone. For most, then, definitive therapy warrants consideration for carotid endarterectomy.

Carotid endarterectomy is a technically challenging operation requiring significant skills in operative and anesthetic techniques. This procedure requires that the surgeon be capable of performing the operation safely and with a stroke rate of 3% or less. Surgeons should perform a sufficient number of these operations per year to maintain procedural skills. In addition, each surgeon should be aware of his or her results.

Indications and Contraindications

Indications for carotid endarterectomy are as follows:

- Symptomatic patients (with TIAs or previous strokes with stable minor deficit), with any

hemodynamically significant lesion (greater than 75% stenosis)
- Good-risk patients with asymptomatic stenosis (at least 75%) (controversial but supported by results of the Asymptomatic Carotid Atherosclerosis Study [ACAS])
- Asymptomatic patients with ulcerated lesions (even with less than 75% stenosis)
- Patients undergoing coronary revascularization with coexistent systematic severe carotid stenosis (controversial)
- Patients with stable neurologic deficits and significant recovery after stroke (advisable to wait 2 to 6 weeks after the initial event)

Contraindications to endarterectomy include profound stroke in evolution and total carotid occlusion. Occlusion that occurs in the early postoperative period, however, is felt to be secondary to technical error and requires a prompt return to the operating room to evacuate the clot and restore the flow before neurologic deficits progress.

Procedure

Carotid endarterectomy involves cross-clamping the proximal common carotid artery and the distal internal and extreme carotid arteries in the neck. The common carotid and internal carotid arteries are then opened longitudinally, and the atheroma is dissected out. The arteriotomy is then closed, and the clamps are removed.

PEARL: Some surgeons use electroencephalographic (EEG) monitoring during cross-clamping or measure distal carotid stump pressures (greater than 25 mm Hg is acceptable) to determine the need for shunting. Other surgeons prefer to perform carotid endarterectomies under local anesthesia with sedation to assess for the development of neurologic symptoms after carotid clamps are applied.

CONTROVERSY: The most prudent practice may be to place a shunt in every case. In this way, endarterectomy can proceed at a controlled pace and allow attention to technical details.

Postoperative Follow-up

In the immediate postoperative period, patients are examined and followed up for any change in speech, vision, and motor function. In addition, cranial nerves IX, X, XII, and the lowest branches of VII are at risk for injury during carotid endarterectomy. Therefore, the patient should be examined for deviation of the tongue, hoarseness, difficulty swallowing, Horner's syndrome, and lip droop. Most surgeons maintain the patients on aspirin. Patients may be discharged 24 hours after carotid endarterectomy.

6
PART

Pediatric Surgery

37
CHAPTER

General Principles of Pediatric Surgery

The care of the surgical infant and child is a special privilege and responsibility. Children may seem nearly indestructible; yet they are nearly unresuscitatable when serious illness intervenes. The rule of thumb for success on a pediatric surgical rotation is to consult staff for any question, no matter how apparently trivial. **PEARL: It's what you don't know that you don't know that will hurt children.**

This chapter and the next two chapters deal with pediatric surgery and serve as a guide to the general principles in the surgical care of infants and children, as an introduction to the unique disorders of the surgical neonate, and as exposure to the common pediatric surgical emergencies.

Children are divided into several standard categories:

Premature (preemies)	37 weeks postgestational age or less
Neonates	0–1 month
Infants	0–24 months
Toddlers	2–4 years

These divisions are useful because the prevalence of surgical diseases differs in each age group.

HISTORY AND PHYSICAL EXAMINATION

The standard history and physical exam differ for children, but are happily short! The following are samples of important items in the history:

Birth history	2-day-old infant boy born by spontaneous vaginal delivery to a 32-year-old woman (gravida 2, para 2) with gestational diabetes; pregnancy complicated by mild polyhydramnios
Immunizations	Up-to-date or 2 months/4 months completed
Family setting	Single mom, siblings, pets, running water and heat, child seats, bike helmets

Nuances in the physical exam include special examination of the following, with examples:

Weight	
Length	
Head circumference	(normal 33–35 cm)
Fontanel	Bulging, flat, closed (normal <5 cm)
Dysmorphic features	Low-set ears, slanted eyes, cleft palate
Sclera	Nonicteric
Murmurs	Patent ductus

Abdominal contour	Scaphoid (diaphragmatic hernia), upper abdominal distention (duodenal atresia), masses, neuroblastoma. *Note:* The normal newborn liver is palpable 3 cm below the costal margin.
Umbilical cord	2 arteries, 1 vein
Anus	Ectopic or patent
Genitalia	Testes descended. *Note:* Prepuce is not retractable until 4 to 6 months of age.
Extremities	Supernumerary digits

FLUID MANAGEMENT AND NUTRITION

PEARL: The first and most important number to calculate when caring for a child is the maintenance fluid rate. One is often instructed to **give maintenance fluids** or **give maintenance and a half.** The child's weight in kilograms must be known or estimated and recorded so that all fluids and drug doses can be based accordingly.

Realize that maintenance fluid for a 500-g baby is 2 mL per hour! Fluid requirements can be calculated from the following general guidelines:

Newborns
Day 1—10% dextrose in water ($D_{10}W$) at 2 mL/kg/hr
Day 2—D_{10} in 25% normal saline (NS) at 4 mL/kg/hr
All others—D_5 in 25% NS or greater with 20 mEq KCl at:
0–10 kg—100 mL/kg/day
10–20 kg—1000 mL/day + 50 mL/kg for each kg over 10 kg
>20 kg—1500 mL/day + 20 mL/kg for each kg over 20 kg

Electrolytes, glucose, and calcium should be checked at 24 hours of life in the hospitalized newborn and at 12 hours of life in unstable premature infants or other high-risk patients. Calcium and electrolytes often need to be added to IV solutions at this time.

Fluid goals need to be increased by 20% when infants are under phototherapy. Fluid goals should be increased by 50% in babies with third-space losses from abdominal surgery or necrotizing enterocolitis.

Nutritional requirements are much greater in infants and young children than in adults. The child's basal metabolic rate is much higher, supporting the enormous growth and development that occur in the early years. General caloric requirements are listed below. These requirements are increased with surgical stress.

Premature	100 kcal/kg/day
Term neonate	90 kcal/kg/day
Toddlers	80 kcal/kg/day
2–9 years	60–70 kcal/kg/day
10–13 years	50–60 kcal/kg/day
Adolescents	40 kcal/kg/day

PEDIATRIC PHYSIOLOGY

Newborns are obligate nasal breathers, and they breathe with their diaphragms. Preemies may have apnea episodes of up to 10 seconds, called **periodic breathing.** This may be normal, but the infant should be watched closely or placed on an apnea monitor. The normal newborn respiratory rate is 40 to 60 breaths per minute. Heart rate in children also varies with age, as shown in Table 37–1.

PEARL: Tachycardia is the most sensitive indicator of hypovolemia in children. Blood pressure is often maintained until arrest by efficient vasoconstriction. A normal blood pressure is not a reliable indicator of volume status in children. Tachycardia and urine output should be monitored closely.

Table 37–1. NORMAL VITAL SIGNS BY AGE

Age	Heart Rate (beats/min)	Respiratory Rate (breaths/min)	Systolic Blood Pressure (mm Hg)	Urinary Output (mL/ kg/hr)
Preemie	160	50	50	1–2
Full-term	140	40	70	1
0–2 yr	120	30	90	1
2–4 yr	110	20	100	0.5
4–6 yr	100	15–20	100	0.5

Temperature Regulation

Babies are more susceptible to cold stress than are adults and older children. Warming lamps should be used for all neonates for examinations, procedures, and so on. The response of newborns to cold stress is an increase in metabolic rate. A prolonged hypermetabolic state leads to the following:

- Anaerobic breakdown of glycogen
- Depletion of energy stores
- Production of lactic acid
- Progressive metabolic acidosis

Skin temperature should be at least 97.5° F. The rectal temperature of a newborn may be misleading and can be normal in the presence of cold stress. Rectal temperature becomes abnormal only after increased metabolic activity fails to maintain normal core temperature. **PEARL: A full-term infant has approximately 5% of an adult's body weight, but 15% of an adult's surface area.**

Premature and Large Newborns

The premature infant is 37 weeks postgestational age or less. High-birth-weight infants (4000 g or more) are considered large for gestational age (LGA). These infants have a high incidence of association with diabetic mothers. Following is a list of the various risks of premature and LGA babies:

Premature
  Apnea
  Hyperbilirubinemia
  Hypocalcemia
  Hypoglycemia
  Hypothermia
  Intracranial hemorrhage
  Respiratory distress syndrome
  Retrolental fibroplasia
  Sepsis
LGA
  Birth injury
  Congenital anomalies
  Hypocalcemia
  Hypoglycemia

Respiration

Respiratory assistance is often required in surgical infants. Premature lungs are highly sensitive to damage from high peak inspiratory pressure. Bronchopulmonary dysplasia and chronic lung disease are the unfortunate sequelae of prolonged ventilation in premature infants. Similarly, blindness can result from retrolental fibroplasia secondary to high fraction of inspired oxygen (FiO_2). Newborn respiratory status is satisfactory if:

- PaO_2 is greater than 60 mm Hg on room air or PaO_2 is greater than 50 mm Hg on 40% to 50% oxygen without an increasing $PaCO_2$.

Respiratory assistance is needed if:

- pH is less than 7.25, PaO_2 is less than 50 torr despite supplemental O_2
- $PaCO_2$ increases into 65-torr range.

Various modes of respiratory assistance are available for newborns. Management options include the isolette for oxygen concentration of less than 30%, and nasal prongs or a head tent for oxygen requirements of 25 to 30%. Continuous positive airway pressure (CPAP) was first described for infants and can provide support of an FiO_2 of 40%. After these levels, mechanical ventilation must be used. All infants undergo time-cycled, pressure-limited mechanical ventilation because of the small tidal volumes involved. Table 37–2 lists standard ventilator settings.

Table 37–2. VENTILATOR SETTINGS FOR INFANTS

Parameter	Setting
Peak inspiratory pressure	16–20
End expiratory pressure	0–4
Positive end-expiratory pressure	3–5
Flow rate	6–10 L/min
Rate (breaths/min)	20–40
FiO_2	23–100%

When weaning from respiratory support, reduce O_2 concentration first unless pressures are excessively high, and reduce the rate to the standard 20–40 range (if it has been higher) before reducing pressure. Patients are generally extubated from a peak inspiratory pressure of 10 to 14.

Infection

Symptoms of infection in infants are often vague and nonspecific. Apnea and bradycardia, tachypnea, lethargy, poor suck, refusal or intolerance of feedings, hypothermia, gastric retention, abdominal distention, cyanosis, and jaundice all suggest infection. **PEARL: Temperature instability rather than temperature maximum is an indicator of sepsis in the neonate.** A white blood cell (WBC) count of 15,000 to 20,000 is normal at birth. The following WBC counts are indicative of sepsis in an infant:

Age	WBCs
1 week	<4000 or >25,000
1 month	<4000 or >15,000
2 months	<4000 or >10,000

The common organisms responsible for neonatal sepsis include:

- β-Hemolytic streptococcus
- *Escherichia coli*
- *Klebsiella*
- *Enterococcus*
- *Pseudomonas*
- *Proteus*
- *Staphylococcus aureus*

Newborns are functionally immunosuppressed and have only maternal antibodies until they are three months of age.

Management

Aggressive management should be instituted in all newborns with signs of infection.

- Patients must be cultured with blood, urine, cerebrospinal fluid, stool, and tracheal swabs.
- Broad-spectrum antibiotics (usually ampicillin and gentamicin or a cephalosporin) should be started.
- Vancomycin and gentamicin are commonly used if there is a risk of methicillin-resistant *Staphylococcus aureus* (MRSA) infection.

Hematology

In the newborn, hematocrit (HCT) and hemoglobin (Hgb) values on cord blood are normally less than on capillary blood. A normal newborn HCT is 40% to 50%, and the patient is not polycythemic until Hgb is greater than 23 or HCT is greater than 70%. At these levels, phlebotomy with plasma volume replacement is considered. Physiologic anemia occurs in infants of 10 to 12 weeks of age, when Hgb drops to 10 g (7 to 8 g at 8 weeks for preemies).

Although most infants with congenital deficiencies of the coagulation factors do not bleed during the first weeks of life, all the coagulation defects may manifest with hemorrhage in the newborn period.

Management of bleeding disorders is guided by the clinical setting and consists of use of the following as needed:

- Platelet transfusions—usually 1 unit/5 kg body weight
- Fresh frozen plasma (FFP)—5 to 10 mL/kg
- Factor replacement as needed

Bilirubin

Hyperbilirubinemia is a problem unique to newborns. Physiologic jaundice occurs in healthy full-term babies. It peaks at three to four days and is generally gone by day seven. Pathologic jaundice is suspected under the following circumstances:

- When jaundice appears within the first 24 hours of life
- When jaundice persists for longer than 10 days

PEARL: Physiologic jaundice is always indirect hyperbilirubinemia. Direct hyperbilirubinemia can be caused by the following:

- Hepatitis of infectious origin (viral origin, rubella, echovirus, coxsackievirus, herpesvirus, toxoplasmosis)
- Biliary obstruction (atresia, bile plug, cyst)
- Hyperalimentation
- Erythroblastosis fetalis
- Metabolic diseases (Wilson's disease, α_1-antitrypsin, galactosemia, tyrosinemia, Niemann-Pick disease, Gaucher's disease, paucity of intrahepatic biliary ducts)

Table 37–3. RECOMMENDED MAXIMAL TOTAL SERUM BILIRUBIN CONCENTRATIONS (mg/dL)

Birth Weight (g)	Uncomplicated Course	Complicated Course
Less than 1250	13	10
1250–1499	15	13
1500–1999	17	15
2000–2499	18	17
2500 and up	20	18

Evaluation of hyperbilirubinemia consists of routine blood work, total and direct bilirubin counts, blood typing and Coombs' testing, CBC with reticulocytes, TORCH titers, metabolic screening, and α_1-antitrypsin levels. Imaging studies, kidney, ureter, and bladder studies, ultrasound, and HIDA scan are used to evaluate biliary anatomy for signs of biliary atresia. Phototherapy is begun when hyperbilirubinemia reaches levels indicated in Table 37–3.

PEDIATRIC RESUSCITATION

Normal blood volume in children is dependent on age:

Neonate	85–95 mL/kg (8–10% of body weight)
Infant	75 mL/kg
Toddler	70 mL/kg

PEARL: Shock from blood loss in a neonate is often manifested by bradycardia rather than tachycardia. (That is, decreased blood volume leads to hypoxia, which leads to bradycardia.)

The following represent general guidelines for resuscitative agents.

- Crystalloid administration: Lactated Ringer's 20 mL/kg × 2 doses, then
- Whole blood 10–20 mL/kg
- Packed cells 10 mL/kg
- Colloid administration: Sodium-(Na-)poor albumin 1–2 g/kg/24 hr
- FFP 10–20 mL/kg
- Plasmanate 10 mL/kg

Electrolyte Abnormalities

Hyponatremia (salt depletion):
(Concentration desired [140] − actual concentration) × 0.6 × kg = mEq Na required (Use 0.7 for infants and children less than 3 years.)

Table 37–4. THE TEN MOST COMMONLY USED PEDIATRIC SURGICAL DRUGS*

Drug	Neonatal <2000 g	Pediatric >2000 g
Ampicillin	50 mg/kg q 12 hr	50 mg/kg q 6 hr
Gentamicin	2 mg/kg q 12 hr	2 mg/kg q 8 hr
Metronidazole (Flagyl)	10 mg/kg q 12 hr	10 mg/kg q 6 hr
Cefazolin	25 mg/kg q 12 hr	25 mg/kg q 6 hr
Morphine	0.1 mg/kg IV	0.1 mg/kg
Codeine	1 mg/kg q 6 hr po	1 mg/kg po
Acetaminophen (Tylenol)	10 mg/kg po	10 mg/kg po
Chloral hydrate		50 mg/kg orally or rectally
Ranitidine (Zantac)		1 mg/kg BID
Metoclopramide (Reglan)		15 mg/kg/dose q 6 hr

*General guidelines only. (Consult your hospital formulary for exact dosages.) Doses listed are IV unless otherwise noted.

Hypokalemia (vomiting)
  KCl 1 mEq/kg IV over 1 hour
Hypoglycemia (glucose < 40)
  25% glucose 2–4 mL/kg IV over 5 minutes, then D15W infusion with gradual reduction to D10W over 48–72 hours
Hypocalcemia (< 7 mg %; normal 8–10 mg% in full-term infants)
  10% calcium gluconate 1 mL/kg over 5 minutes (Avoid extravasation.)
Metabolic acidosis: (pH <7.25)
  Sodium bicarbonate dose = base deficit × 0.3 × kg

Table 37–4 lists the ten most common drugs needed for pediatric surgical care.

38
CHAPTER

The Surgical Neonate

GENERAL PRINCIPLES OF EVALUATION

The care of a neonate requires an alert clinician. Because of the neonate's limited organ system reserve, the status of the neonate can change rapidly.

Four cardinal signs should signal a possible surgical emergency in a newborn:

- Bilious vomiting (yellow or green colored)
- Abdominal distention
- Bloody stool
- Respiratory distress

PEARL: Generally, bilious vomiting in an infant means intestinal obstruction until proven otherwise! Vomiting is usually associated with abdominal distention. However, there may be no distention in the presence of such surgical problems as duodenal atresia, stenosis, annular pancreas, and malrotation with midgut volvulus (twisting). Abdominal distention may be caused by intestinal obstruction, pneumoperitoneum, pseudocysts, ascites, and other problems (Table 38–1).

The most common newborn intra-abdominal mass is due to multicystic kidney or urinary tract obstruction. Intestinal duplication, mesenteric cysts, hydro- or hematocolpos, or intestinal gaseous inflation from ventilator

Table 38–1. COMMON CAUSES OF NEWBORN BOWEL OBSTRUCTION

Mechanical
Intestinal atresia (duodenal, ileal, jejunal, colon),
  pyloric stenosis
Malrotation with midgut volvulus
Meconium ileus (cystic fibrosis)
Small left colon syndrome (diabetic mothers)
Meconium peritonitis (with perforation, adhesions,
  and pseudocyst formation)
Incarcerated hernia (inguinal, diaphragmatic)
Necrotizing enterocolitis
Duplication

Functional
Hirschsprung's disease (aganglionosis)
Paralytic ileus
Sepsis
Peritonitis
Maternal drugs (magnesium, diazepam [Valium], heroin)
Electrolyte abnormalities (hypokalemia,
  hypermagnesemia, uremia)

support and continuous positive airway pressure (CPAP) can also cause abdominal distention.

Bloody stool implies a break in the mucosal lining of the bowel (suspicion of possible necrotizing enterocolitis or volvulus).

Respiratory distress may indicate diaphragmatic hernia or eventration, pneumothorax, pulmonary cyst, cystadenomatoid malformation, congenital heart disease, esophageal atresia or tracheoesophageal fistula, or tracheal abnormality.

Evaluation of the Surgical Abdomen

When evaluating a newborn for a possible intestinal problem, there should be a film of the *full abdomen* including chest (i.e., a "babygram"), as well as a *left lateral decubitus* film (liver side up) to evaluate for free air. If you have only one film, get the decubitus view.

PEARL: In the newborn, it is impossible to determine the position of the colon without a contrast study. Haustral markings are not apparent in the newborn. Intestinal obstruction can often be diagnosed with minimal testing (plain films or contrast studies). Specific types are discussed in greater detail later in this chapter. The following are diagnostic points to keep in mind during evaluation of the neonate:

- Plain x-rays can be useful in identifying a high obstruction with a "double-bubble" sign, suggestive of duodenal atresia or malrotation and volvulus.
- Low obstruction with multiple dilated loops suggests distal jejunal, ileal, or colonic lesions.
- Contrast enema in the setting of bowel obstruction demonstrates a high cecum in malrotation.
- A microcolon suggests small-bowel atresia, meconium ileus, or long-segment Hirschsprung's disease.
- A dilated colon can be associated with Hirschsprung's disease, or meconium plug.

There are only a few true emergencies in which a baby requires immediate operation:

- Suspected malrotation with midgut volvulus
- Pneumoperitoneum (due to perforated viscus)
- Gastroschisis
- Ruptured omphalocele

Management

Initial management procedures are the same for most neonatal surgical conditions:
1. Resuscitate infant.

   - Correct shock, dehydration, electrolyte, and acid-base abnormalities.
   - Intubate and give respiratory support if needed.
   - Keep infant warm.
2. Secure IV access.
3. Insert nasogastric tube.
4. Give vitamin K.
5. Obtain baseline blood studies: electrolytes, CBC, type and crossmatch, bilirubin, glucose.

6. Administer antibiotics.
7. Obtain preoperative x-rays: barium enema, abdominal ultrasound.
8. Talk to family and obtain permission to operate.

CONDITIONS OF OBSTRUCTION

Duodenal Atresia

Duodenal atresia is a complete obstruction of the duodenum thought to be caused by recanalization failure of the proliferated duodenal mucosa at 5 to 6 weeks gestation. It represents about half of all intestinal atresias and is associated with Down syndrome 30% of the time. Half of patients with duodenal atresia are low-birthweight infants, and many have associated malrotation.

Presenting symptoms include maternal polyhydramnios, bilious vomiting, and feeding intolerance. The classic x-ray appearance is that of the **double-bubble.** In 85% of patients, the obstruction is distal to Vater's papilla (ampulla of Vater), but in 15% the obstruction is proximal and vomiting is therefore nonbilious.

Differential diagnosis includes annular pancreas and malrotation.

Treatment of duodenal atresia is surgical duodenoduodenostomy. Surgery is emergent if malrotation cannot be ruled out (by barium enema).

Small-Bowel Atresias

Small-bowel atresia is complete obstruction of the small bowel, thought to be caused by vascular occlusion with aseptic necrosis. This may be due to defects in the mesenteric arcade or intrauterine volvulus. Associated anomalies are uncommon.

Symptoms include maternal polyhydramnios, bilious vomiting, and abdominal distention. X-rays can be diagnostic with multiple dilated loops, air-fluid levels, and no distal air. Barium enema, if obtained, reveals a microcolon due to disuse. **PEARL: Bowel gas should be seen throughout the intestine by 24 hours of life in a normal newborn.**

Small-bowel atresia may occur in a variety of patterns. The details are beyond our scope (refer to a formal surgical text).

Imperforate Anus

Imperforate anus represents the most distal bowel atresia. It usually occurs in male infants (3:2) and can range from simply a thin membrane covering the anal verge to a high rectal atresia associated with a urogenital fistula.

Diagnosis is made by physical examination and failure to pass meconium. The presence of associated anomalies is high (from 30% to 60%), and imperforate anus is part of **VATER syndrome**. VACTRL or VATER syndrome includes:

Vertebral anomalies
Anal atresia
Cardiac anomalies
Tracheo**E**sophageal fistula
Renal anomalies
Limb abnormalities

Workup should include cardiac, renal, and perineal ultrasound.

Treatment of imperforate anus consists of perineal anoplasty for low lesions and posterior sagittal anorectoplasty (PSARP) for high lesions.

Malrotation and Midgut Volvulus

Malrotation results from failure of proper re-entrance and fixation of intestines from the extraembryonic coelom during week six in utero with resultant abnormal intestinal position and attachments. The cecum normally resides in the right lower quadrant with proper rotation and fixation. With failure of rotation, the mesenteric root is narrow, and fixation is around only the superior mesenteric vessels. This anatomic arrangement leads to the potential for midgut volvulus, and intestinal strangulation.

Malrotation is associated occasionally with duodenal atresia, usually with diaphragmatic hernia, and always with omphalocele and gastroschisis. The duodenum and small intestine lie to the right of the spine, whereas the cecum and colon reside in the right upper quadrant or midabdomen.

Diagnostic Findings

Symptoms of malrotation in the acute setting include bilious vomiting, often initially with a scaphoid, benign appearing abdomen. **PEARL: Bilious vomiting in an infant is malrotation until proven otherwise!** Most patients have onset of symptoms in the first week of life (usually the first three days), with volvulus reported in up to 85% of the babies presenting in infancy.

Chronic malrotation is due to Ladd's bands or intermittent volvulus and presents with cyclic abdominal pain, bilious vomiting, or malabsorption. **Ladd's bands** are the fibrous bands that extend from the abnormally positioned cecum to the right upper quadrant. They often cross the duodenum, causing proximal obstruction.

The following are typical test results in infants with malrotation:

- X-rays reveal duodenal obstruction with a dilated stomach, and near gasless abdomen.
- Upper gastrointestinal series demonstrates an absent ligament of Treitz with a coiled spring appearance to the duodenum.
- Barium enema shows the cecum in the upper abdomen.

The differential diagnosis of malrotation includes duodenal atresia and annular pancreas.

Treatment

The following are procedure guidelines for surgical treatment of an infant with malrotation:

- Emergency laparotomy is done by means of a supraumbilical transverse incision when malrotation is diagnosed or unable to be ruled out.
- The volvulus is reduced in a counterclockwise manner.

- Ladd's bands are divided.
- The mesentery is widened, thus placing the small bowel in the right abdomen and the large bowel in the left abdomen.
- Appendectomy is always performed to prevent future error in diagnosis.

PEARL: Gangrenous loss of small bowel with resultant short-gut syndrome is one of the greatest tragedies in pediatric surgery.

ABDOMINAL WALL DEFECTS

Omphalocele and Gastroschisis

Omphalocele and gastroschisis are the two common congenital abdominal wall defects. The overall incidence is about 1 in 5000 live births. Although the treatment is similar, the two defects have many differences, as shown in Table 38–2.

DISORDERS ASSOCIATED WITH MECONIUM

Meconium Ileus

Meconium ileus is the most common of the three newborn disorders associated with meconium. It is characterized by distal small-bowel obstruction secondary to solid meconium concretions. Most patients who present with meconium ileus have cystic fibrosis (the condition occurs in about 15% of patients with cystic fibrosis).

Patients with meconium ileus present with abdominal distention, bilious vomiting, and a doughy-feeling abdomen. Often, meconium-filled loops of bowel are palpable. The rectum is often devoid of meconium.

PEARL: Sweat chloride or genetic testing is mandatory in patients with meconium ileus (to rule out cystic fibrosis). Radiographs reveal a characteristic "soap-suds" or "ground-glass" appearance, representing meconium mixed with air.

Table 38–2. COMPARISON OF OMPHALOCELE AND GASTROSCHISIS

	Omphalocele	Gastroschisis
Cause	Failure of umbilical fusion of the mesenchymal abdominal wall folds at 10 weeks' gestation	In utero rupture of a cord hernia, possibly during normal migration of the bowel out of the abdominal cavity
Covering	Covered with an amnion and peritoneal sac	No covering
Position of defect	Middle of umbilicus with cord usually inferior to defect	Right side of umbilicus with cord to the left
Associated anomalies	Common (> 50%), including cardiac, renal, and chromosomal anomalies; Beckwith-Weideman syndrome	Rare Mostly associated atresias (10–15%), likely secondary to mechanical disruption of mesenteric vasculature
Malrotation	Yes	Yes
Treatment	Primary closure, if possible, or placement of a temporary Silastic "silo" with gradual reduction of abdominal viscera over 5–7 days, followed by closure Difficult abdominal wall closure in giant (>5 cm) defects	Same
Complications		Prolonged ileus common
Mortality	Primarily dependent on associated anomalies	<10%

Initial treatment of choice for meconium ileus is non-operative with meglumine diatrizoate (Gastrografin) enemas. Operation is indicated if enemas fail to clear the obstruction (50% success rate) or if the diagnosis is in doubt.

Meconium Peritonitis

Meconium peritonitis is a sign of intrauterine bowel perforation. Sterile intra-abdominal meconium leads to an intense inflammatory response, resulting in intra-abdominal calcification of meconium. Calcifications on plain film are a contraindication to contrast enema, and most babies require laparotomy.

Some infants with meconium peritonitis can be very ill with significant fluid sequestration. Others simply present with a large meconium pseudocyst.

Meconium Plug Syndrome

Meconium plug syndrome is a colonic obstruction with inspissated meconium. The cause is unclear. Babies present with abdominal distention and failure to pass meconium. Contrast enema is diagnostic and is often therapeutic, demonstrating a small left colon with a proximally dilated colon filled with meconium. This diagnosis can be difficult to differentiate from Hirschsprung's disease, and rectal biopsy is recommended.

DISORDERS OF MALDEVELOPMENT AND PREMATURITY

Hirschsprung's Disease

Hirschsprung's disease, also known as **aganglionic megacolon,** results from developmental arrest in the migration of ganglion cells from neural crest tissue to the bowel. Ganglion cells are absent from both the myenteric (Auerbach's) and the submucosal (Meissner's) plexuses. This results in spastic tonic contraction of bowel with proximally dilated obstructed bowel.

Of the infants affected, 85% are boys, and about 5% of the cases are familial. Hirschsprung's disease is associated with multiple endocrine neoplasia type II (MEN II) and also with Down syndrome. No skip lesions are found in patients with Hirschsprung's disease. Eighty percent have involvement to the level of the rectosigmoid, 10% have involvement to the splenic flexure, and 10% have aganglionosis affecting the total colon or more proximal bowel.

Hirschsprung's disease is rare in premature infants. In full-term babies, it usually manifests at birth with abdominal distention and failure to pass meconium. **PEARL: Of normal babies, 75% pass meconium in the first 24 hours of life; 90% pass meconium by 48 hours.**

Diagnosis of Hirschsprung's disease is suggested by barium enema revealing a contracted rectum with proximal dilatation and failure to evacuate the barium within 24 hours. Definitive diagnosis is made by rectal biopsy demonstrating absence of ganglion cells.

Treatment is colostomy with subsequent "pull-through" procedures.

CONTROVERSY: Some centers advocate primary pull-through procedures without prior colostomy.

- **Swenson's**—removal of the aganglionic rectum followed by a primary anastomosis between healthy colon and the anal verge
- **Duhamel**—retention of the anterior region of the aganglionic rectum, which is anastomosed to the posterior and pulled through healthy bowel, creating a rectal pouch
- **Soave**—also known as an endorectal pull-through, in which proximal normal bowel is brought through the aganglionic rectum, which has been stripped of its abnormal mucosa

Overall survival rate is 90%, with deaths occurring from fulminant Hirschsprung's enterocolitis.

Necrotizing Enterocolitis

Necrotizing enterocolitis (NEC) is a disease of prematurity. **PEARL: NEC is now a leading cause of death in**

premature infants. NEC is characterized by ischemic necrosis of the gastrointestinal tract, leading to perforation. The exact cause is unclear; however, NEC is often associated with the stressed premature infant (respiratory distress syndrome, sepsis, and cardiac disease).

Signs of NEC include abdominal distention, feeding intolerance with bilious aspirates, bloody stools, lethargy, temperature instability, and new apneic and bradycardiac episodes. Diagnosis is confirmed by abdominal radiographs showing pneumatosis (gas within the intestinal wall), portal vein gas, or free air.

Unless there is evidence of perforation, initial treatment of patients with NEC is nonoperative. Patients receive bowel rest with nasogastric decompression, IV hydration, and broad-spectrum antibiotic coverage for 14 days. Patients are followed closely with frequent (every 6 to 8 hours) abdominal exams and x-rays.

Indications for operation for NEC are those of transmural bowel necrosis, consisting of the following:

- Abdominal tenderness
- Abdominal wall erythema
- Persistent obstruction
- A fixed loop of bowel on serial x-rays or free intra-abdominal air signifying perforation.

Surgical treatment involves resecting the dead bowel and creating temporary ostomies. The most significant long-term complication of NEC is short bowel syndrome. Overall mortality rate of patients with NEC is about 25%.

CONDITIONS OF RESPIRATORY DISTRESS

Tracheoesophageal Fistula and Esophageal Atresia

Of the surgical causes of respiratory distress in the newborn, tracheal esophageal fistula (TEF) is the most common. Esophageal atresia (EA; blind-ending esophagus) and TEF (connection to trachea) develop in the third to sixth week of fetal life when the trachea and esophagus develop and then separate from the foregut. Table 38–3 shows the five types and their frequency.

Table 38–3. TYPES OF ESOPHAGEAL ATRESIA (EA)

Name	Description	Percentage of Cases
Type A	EA with no TEF (pure atresia)	7%
Type B	EA with proximal fistula	1%
Type C	EA with distal TEF	85%
Type D	EA with both proximal and distal TEF	3%
Type E	TEF with no EA (H-type)	4%

TEF = tracheal esophageal fistula.

The presenting symptom is most often excessive salivation. However, symptoms range from difficulty with feeding to frank respiratory distress due to air preferentially entering the stomach through a large fistula. The diagnosis is commonly made when the nasogastric tube is unable to be passed.

X-ray reveals the nasogastric tube coiled in the proximal pouch. Air in the gastrointestinal tract signals the presence of a fistula from the trachea to the distal esophagus.

Treatment

Initial management in the stable patient is directed toward preventing aspiration.

Following are principles of treatment for the patient with TEF/EA:

- A sump tube is placed in the pouch, and the patient is positioned upright to prevent reflux of gastric contents up the fistula into the lungs.
- Antibiotics are given.
- An x-ray is taken to evaluate pouch length.
- An echocardiogram is obtained to rule out associated cardiac anomalies and assess the position of the aortic arch.
- The patient then undergoes surgery with separation of the distal esophagus from the trachea, clo-

sure of the trachea, and primary anastomosis of the esophageal ends.

- In the premature patient or the patient in respiratory distress, emergent surgery may be required to ligate the fistula.

Overall survival and prognosis for patients with this lesion are excellent.

Congenital Diaphragmatic Hernia

Congenital diaphragmatic hernia (CDH) occurs during the 8th to 12th week of gestation if the diaphragm fails to form completely. This incomplete development allows abdominal contents to herniate into the chest cavity. The resultant pulmonary hypoplasia, resulting from mass effect in the chest preventing lung growth, carries a high mortality rate (50%).

The most common type of CDH is the **Bochdalek hernia** with a posterolateral defect. The **Morgagni anterior parasternal hernia** is relatively rare.

Patients present with severe respiratory distress. Patients have associated malrotation, and cardiac defects are found in 10% to 20%.

Treatment

The current approach to management is *immediate intubation* (eliminating mask ventilation with further gaseous distention of bowel), *nasogastric decompression, IV hydration*, and *stabilization*.

Patients are treated medically for pulmonary hypertension, and repair of the diaphragmatic defect is delayed. Medical stabilization and control of pulmonary hypertension may require extraordinary measures, such as nitric oxide therapy, partial liquid ventilation, and ECMO (extracorporeal membrane oxygenation) cardiopulmonary bypass.

Despite intensive therapy, overall severe morbidity and mortality remains 40 to 50%, prompting investigators to explore fetal therapies to prevent the pulmonary hypoplasia.

CONTROVERSY: The management of diaphragmatic hernia remains controversial in all aspects.

39

The Surgical Child

COMMON PEDIATRIC SURGICAL PROBLEMS

This chapter focuses on common problems associated with pediatric patients in the emergency room and on the pediatric wards. Emphasis is on tips to facilitate initial patient management.

Intestinal Obstruction

Pediatric surgical problems generally present as some form of intestinal obstruction. The differential diagnosis can be simplified by dividing into age groups:

Infants and toddlers
  Pyloric stenosis
  Incarcerated inguinal hernias
  Intussusception
  Hirschsprung's disease
  Malrotation with midgut volvulus
Toddlers and up
  Appendicitis
  Incarcerated hernia
  Meckel's diverticulum (gastrointestinal bleeding)
  Tumors
  Malrotation with midgut volvulus

PEARL: Bilious vomiting in a child is malrotation until proven otherwise! Although malrotation with midgut volvulus is the most dreaded diagnosis, the most common cause of bowel obstruction in children is incarcerated hernia. A complete physical examination remains the mainstay of diagnosis of intestinal obstruction.

Acute Appendicitis

The most common request for consultation of a surgical resident is "abdominal pain—rule out appendicitis." **PEARL: Appendicitis is the most common condition in children requiring intra-abdominal surgery.** The pediatric peak incidence for this disorder is in the mid-teens. It is less common in children under 3 years, but not rare.

The tempo of appendicitis is much faster in children than in older people. Appendicitis runs a more rapid and deadly course in children, with perforation occurring within 6 to 12 hours of onset of symptoms in the very young. Other differences in children with appendicitis include the following:

- Poor localization and walling off
- More rapid progression of disease with early systemic toxicity (fever, vomiting, diarrhea, and dehydration)
- 60 to 70% perforation rate in children under 4 years

Diagnostic Findings

The common symptoms of appendicitis are pain, fever, and vomiting. Pain is almost always the first symptom, often poorly localized in children. It usually precedes vomiting except in very young children, who may not complain of pain. **PEARL: Localized point tenderness, when present, is the cardinal sign in appendicitis.** Fever is usually 100° to 101°F.

PEARL: Fever of 104°F or higher without signs of peritonitis and early in the course makes one hesitate to diagnose acute appendicitis. (Think "pneumonia.")

White blood cell count is almost always over 10,000; x-rays are often nonspecific. Suggestive findings on x-ray are right lower quadrant mass effect, localized ileus, and fecolith.

Chest x-ray is most important. Pneumonia can present with abdominal pain in young children.

Differential diagnosis of acute appendicitis includes the following:

Pneumonia	Ruptured ovarian cyst
Gastroenteritis	Twisted ovary
Constipation	Mittelschmerz
Mesenteric adenitis	Pelvic inflammatory
Hemolytic-uremic syndrome (HUS)	disease
Henoch-Schönlein purpura (HSP) (check for rash, urinalysis, and platelets)	Testicular torsion
	Epididymitis
	Urinary tract infection
	Ureteral stones

Treatment

Management of children with acute appendicitis involves the following:

- IV hydration via 20 mL/kg bolus over 30 minutes, then twice the maintenance rate.
- Antibiotics are given when a decision to operate is made. Single broad-spectrum coverage is used if early appendicitis is suspected, or triple antibiotics if perforation is suspected.
- Foley catheter and nasogastric tube are used for the seriously ill.
- Postoperatively, IV fluids are given at 1 1/2 to 2 times the maintenance rate, and antibiotics are given for 7 to 10 days if perforated appendicitis.

Pyloric Stenosis

Pyloric stenosis is hypertrophy and hyperplasia of the pyloric musculature, causing gastric outlet obstruction. The exact cause is unknown. Its peak incidence is at two to six weeks of age, and it occurs more commonly in male infants than in females (4:1), typically first-born boys.

Diagnostic Findings

Symptoms are of progressive nonbilious vomiting of undigested formula. Mothers often describe "projectile" vomiting, occasionally with blood streaking. Physical examination reveals gastric peristaltic waves on the abdomen. **PEARL: In a relaxed patient, the pyloric mass can be felt as a "palpable olive" in the epigastrium.** The dehydrated patient may have a sunken fontanel.

Today with increased awareness of the disorder, patients rarely present with severe dehydration, but the classic electrolyte abnormality of hypochloremic, hypokalemic metabolic alkalosis is still seen. Associated paradoxical aciduria is less common, but mild hyperbilirubinemia is commonly seen.

If the diagnosis cannot be definitively made by physical examination, then either upper gastrointestinal series (UGI) or ultrasound can be used. UGI shows a "string sign" or "double-track" sign with visible pyloric "shoulders." Ultrasound, which requires an experienced pediatric radiologist, is positive when the pylorus shows more than 4 mm in wall thickness and more than 14 mm in length.

The differential diagnosis of pyloric stenosis includes:

- Gastroesophageal reflux
- Duodenal web
- Duodenal stenosis
- Duplication

Treatment

PEARL: Pyloric stenosis is a medical emergency, not a surgical emergency. The most important aspect of management is correction of fluid and electrolyte imbalances. IV hydration is begun with a bolus 10 mL/kg normal saline followed by 1½ maintenance rate 5% dextrose/normal saline (D_5/NS) solution. Fluids are changed to D_5 1/2NS + 20 mEq potassium chloride (KCl) when electrolytes are known, and urine output is restored. Potassium deficits are corrected. Nasogastric tubes are not needed, but the patient is given nothing by mouth (NPO). The infant is ready for surgery when fluid and electrolyte status is corrected.

Preoperatively, metabolic alkalosis must be corrected (bicarbonate<30) to prevent postoperative hypoventilation and a compensatory respiratory acidosis.

The surgeon should be present at induction to ensure that the infant's stomach is aspirated before giving anesthesia. A classic pyloromyotomy (Ramstedt's operation) is definitive surgical treatment.

Postoperatively, feeds usually begin in six hours with small amounts of Pedialyte and are advanced slowly over the next 24 hours in both concentration and volume on a two- to three-hourly basis. Patients are discharged on postoperative day one or two, with the mother reassured that some early vomiting is to be expected.

Intussusception

Intussusception, the prolapse of one portion of the intestine into an adjoining part, is a disease of infancy. Infants under one year of age make up 80% of cases with a peak incidence at 5 to 7 months. Male infants are affected more than female infants (2:1). Eighty percent of cases are ileocolic; 15% are ileoileal.

The cause is unknown or idiopathic in 90 to 95% of cases of infantile intussusception. Rarely, a Meckel's diverticulum, polyp, duplication, or hematoma from HSP can be the inciting cause. In patients over 2 years old, small bowel tumors such as lymphomas are more commonly associated.

Symptoms are that of a healthy child with sudden episodes of severe abdominal pain, vomiting, and later "currant jelly" stools. The child may also present with lethargy, diarrhea, and vomiting. Abdominal exam is variable. The abdomen may be soft, have a mass in the right upper quadrant with an empty right lower quadrant, or be distended with diffuse tenderness.

PEARL: Plain films cannot rule out intussusception. Plain films may show obstruction or a paucity of gas in the colon.

Treatment

The treatment of intussusception involves attempts at reduction with barium or air enema if the child has no toxic symptoms and no peritonitis. Before being administered the enema, patients must have a surgical evaluation, IV hydration, and antibiotic coverage (usually a second-generation cephalosporin).

If the reduction is successful, the child is admitted with IV hydration at 1½ times the maintenance rate. The patient is kept NPO until he or she passes gas and the abdomen is soft. Recurrence rate after enema is 5 to 7 percent.

If reduction fails, the patient needs urgent operation. At surgery, a transverse right lower quadrant (some use low right upper quadrant) incision is used. Manual reduction of the intussusceptus is performed with a push—not a pull—technique. Appendectomy is always performed, and resection is reserved for gangrenous bowel or severe serosal disruption. Recurrence rate after surgery is 2 percent.

Meckel's Diverticulum

A Meckel's diverticulum is the remnant of the omphalomesenteric duct (or vitelline duct), which connects the primitive midgut to the yolk sac in the embryo. It is a true diverticulum containing all layers of the bowel wall. A Meckel's diverticulum is generally found 50 to 90 cm proximal to the ileocecal valve on the antimesenteric border of the ileum. It is three times more common in boys than in girls.

Typical presentation is sudden painless bleeding in the toddler age group (50% of patients), but intestinal obstruction can be a manifestation in an older age group (25%), as well as inflammation mimicking appendicitis (<20%). Bleeding is the result of ectopic mucosa (gastric in 85% of cases), causing ulceration of the adjacent ileal mucosa.

The incidence of Meckel's diverticulum is approximately 3% in autopsy specimens. Ninety percent of affected patients are asymptomatic. **PEARL: Resection is *not* done routinely when Meckel's diverticulum is found incidentally at laparotomy for another indication.**

Diagnosis of Meckel's diverticulum can be made by a positive technetium pertechnetate scan or "Meckel's scan," which demonstrates a focus of contrast indicating gastric mucosa in an area outside of the stomach. **PEARL: Meckel's diverticular disease can be remembered by the "rule of twos."**

2 years old
2 inches in length
2% incidence in population
2 feet from the ileocecal valve
2% are symptomatic
2 times more common in boys

Treatment is surgical resection.

Thyroglossal Duct Cyst

A thyroglossal duct cyst is a midline cystic mass usually located 1 cm below the hyoid. It is a remnant of thyroglossal duct, which extends from the foramen cecum as a midline diverticulum from the pharyngeal floor. The duct passes through the hyoid bone.

Thyroglossal duct cysts should be excised when diagnosed. The cyst may be solid and consist of functioning thyroid tissue in 5% of cases. **PEARL: Preoperative thyroid scan should be done if normal thyroid gland cannot be clearly felt.**

Branchial Cleft Cysts and Sinuses

Branchial cleft anomalies are most often found in the lateral neck. They are epithelial-lined remnants of the primitive branchial clefts, which connect to the skin of the anterior neck. Cleft cysts (most common) and sinuses are located in the submandibular area. Approximately 30% of these cysts end blindly.

Enlarged Lymph Nodes

Palpable lymph nodes are common in children. They usually represent chronic lymphadenitis. Any solitary, firm, discrete, nontender node deserves consideration for excision. If the node is not smaller over a period of observation, excision should be recommended.

Differential diagnosis includes Hodgkin's lymphoma, thyroid neoplasm, atypical mycobacteria, and cat-scratch fever.

Cystic Hygromas

Cystic hygromas are congenital malformations of lymphatics. Most occur in the cervical area, but they are seen in almost all areas of the body. Total surgical excision is the treatment of choice. It is important to attempt entire removal, but not at the expense of sacrificing nerves and other critical structures.

Torticollis

In the newborn infant, torticollis is a neck mass situated in the sternocleidomastoid muscle, which can appear in an infant between one and three weeks of age. This represents hemorrhage and fibrosis of the muscle body. There is usually a history of difficult birth (breech presentation or forceps delivery).

Diagnosis can be confirmed by cervical ultrasound. Differential diagnosis includes a cervical teratoma, cervical neuroblastoma, or a soft tissue tumor, such as a rhabdomyosarcoma (very unusual).

Treatment is with physical therapy and stretching exercises.

Hemangioma

Hemangiomas are common newborn vascular malformations. Most require no treatment. A hemangioma is frequently noted at 2 to 3 weeks after birth with gradual growth to about 1 year of age. It then undergoes spontaneous regression and disappearance over the next few years.

Therapy may be indicated for rapidly growing facial lesions and for large lesions with platelet trapping.

α-Interferon has shown clinical promise. Surgery is occasionally required for cosmetically disfiguring lesions that do not regress over several years' time.

Breast Lesions

Neonatal breast lesions represent physiologic hypertrophy due to circulating maternal hormones. In prepubertal patients, these lesions represent physiologic hypertrophy of unknown cause. Breast lesions can appear in boys and girls and usually disappear when the infant is 6 to 12 months old. **PEARL: Do not excise or biopsy breast lesions in girls!**

Fibroadenoma is the most common breast tumor after puberty. It is a firm, rubbery, discrete mass and should be excised if large (>2 cm) (see Chapter 8). Cystic disease and carcinoma are extremely rare under 18 years of age.

Caustic Ingestion

Caustic injury due to ingestion of strong alkali (e.g., soap powders, drain-opening liquids, lye) or acid (rare) is not uncommon in children. **PEARL: Most caustic injuries occur only to the lips and oral pharynx, but esophageal damage must always be ruled out.** Infants tend to drink liquids in bolus "gulps," and thus material can traverse the oral pharynx and damage the esophagus.

Most commercial soap powders and liquids do not contain enough alkali (hypochlorite) to do any damage. However, inhalation of concentrated soap powders can cause significant oral and tracheal burns.

Signs and Symptoms

Symptoms of caustic injury include drooling, refusal to swallow, and pain.

Respiratory distress due to laryngeal swelling is always a major concern in the first 12 hours after caustic ingestion. Tachycardia, fever, and abdominal pain are early signs of possible full-thickness necrosis (thorax or abdomen).

Chest x-rays can show aspiration, pleural effusion, or mediastinal air. Esophageal swallow or contrast study is usually obtained at seven days in cases of severe burns as a baseline study. Obtain a water-contrast study earlier if full-thickness necrosis and possible perforation are suspected.

Treatment

All patients with suspected caustic injuries are admitted for observation. Children with burns of the lips or oral pharynx are kept NPO and given IV hydration. If the pharynx is free of burns and the infant is swallowing normally with no drooling after 12 hours, consider starting oral fluids. Esophagoscopy is not mandatory. If there is any question as to the severity of injury, esophagoscopy is indicated.

Children with pharyngeal burns or severe burns are admitted to the pediatric intensive care unit, and elective intubation is considered if respiratory symptoms develop. Patients are kept NPO, and IV hydration and broad-spectrum antibiotics are given. Esophagoscopy is performed within 24 hours after these burns. If extensive or severe burns are found, a subclavian line for total parenteral nutrition or a gastrostomy for feedings and dilation is inserted.

Choledochal Cyst

Choledochal cysts are cystic enlargements of the bile ducts. These cysts are seen most frequently in infants and young children, although they can be seen in all age groups. **PEARL: The classic presentation of choledochal cyst is the triad of a right upper quadrant mass, jaundice, and abdominal pain.** There are four common types of choledochal cysts:

Type I	Saccular dilatation of the common hepatic and common bile ducts (most common type)
Type II	A lateral saccular dilatation off the side of the common duct.
Type III	An intraduodenal choledochocele
Type IV	Multiple intrahepatic and extrahepatic cysts

The diagnosis is usually made by ultrasound.

Treatment of choledochal cysts is complete surgical excision when possible, followed by hepaticojejunostomy reconstruction. Complete resection is advocated owing to a long-term risk of cholangiocarcinoma arising from the cyst lining.

PEDIATRIC TUMORS

The most common cancers in childhood are leukemia, lymphoma, and central nervous system tumors. The most common solid tumors that the pediatric surgeon treats are neuroblastoma and Wilms' tumor.

Neuroblastoma

Neuroblastoma is the most common solid tumor of infancy. It occurs in 1 in 10,000 live births. It is an embryonal tumor of neural crest origin and is most commonly found in the adrenal glands (50% of cases). Other common locations include the intra-abdominal parasympathetic ganglia (25%), posterior mediastinum (20%), and the neck and pelvis (5%). Patients with neuroblastomas generally present with an asymptomatic abdominal mass, or the tumor is an incidental finding on chest x-ray obtained for other indications.

Treatment

Treatment is usually a combination of surgery and chemotherapy and depends on the stage and biology of the tumor. DNA ploidy and N-*myc* amplification are useful prognostic indicators. Overall survival is affected by age, with 75% of children under age one surviving. Stage I and stage II tumors are associated with greater than 80% survival; stage III and IV with less than 20%. Bone marrow transplantation is effective for patients with metastatic disease.

Wilms' Tumor

Wilms' tumor is an embryonal tumor of renal origin. There are 500 new cases a year in the United States. Patients with Wilms' tumors are generally toddlers and present with a unilateral asymptomatic abdominal mass. Ten percent of patients have hematuria.

Wilms' tumor is associated with other abnormalities including aniridia, hemihypertrophy, and Beckwith-Wiedemann syndrome (a combination of macroglossia, omphalocele, visceromegaly, and hypoglycemia at birth).

Treatment is surgical resection in stage I and stage II disease and combination therapy in higher stages. The best indicator of survival is the histologic subtype of the tumor, with more than 90% survival rate for lesions with favorable histology.

Index

An "f" following a page number indicates a figure; a "t" following a page number indicates a table.